The Durable Runner

THE DURABLE RUNNER

A Guide to
Injury-Free Running

Alison Heilig

Foreword by Sage Rountree

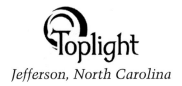

Jefferson, North Carolina

Library of Congress Cataloguing-in-Publication Data

Names: Heilig, Alison, 1980– author.
Title: The durable runner : a guide to injury-free running /
Alison Heilig.
Description: Jefferson, North Carolina : Toplight, 2019 |
Includes bibliographical references and index.
Identifiers: LCCN 2019029381 | ISBN 9781476678337 (paperback) ∞
ISBN 9781476638263 (ebook)
Subjects: LCSH: Running—Training. | Sports injuries—Prevention. |
Running—Physiological aspects.
Classification: LCC GV1061.5 .H445 2019 | DDC 613.7/172—dc23
LC record available at https://lccn.loc.gov/2019029381

British Library cataloguing data are available

ISBN (print) 978-1-4766-7833-7
ISBN (ebook) 978-1-4766-3826-3

Front cover image © 2019 Mike Cadotte, photographer

Printed in the United States of America

Toplight is an imprint of McFarland & Company, Inc., Publishers

*Box 611, Jefferson, North Carolina 28640
www.toplightbooks.com*

For the ones who feel fragile—
things are about to change.

Table of Contents

Acknowledgments

Writing a book often felt like an extraordinarily solitary activity— but I was never truly alone in the process. It took a village to make this project a reality and I'm so proud to say that—as villages go—I truly have been surrounded by one of the best.

To my husband, Chris, thanks for, well … everything. I'm not sure I could ever adequately express how much I appreciate you letting me vent, putting up with the many days and weekends spent at my desk, and most importantly always reminding me that I'm doing my best and that will ultimately be good enough.

To my incredible mom, Karen Hoover, for raising me right, giving me space, and never letting me forget that I had a shoulder to lean on. Thank you for teaching me what it means to face life with grace and durability.

To my teacher and mentor, Sage Rountree, for the push I needed to start this book and the encouragement and wisdom given every step of the way. Without you, I might never have had the guts to go for it, and even if I did, I'd have had absolutely no clue where to even begin. And even if I did, this book would not have made nearly as much sense without your lightning-fast edits and thoughtful feedback on the manuscript.

To my agent, Robert Kern, for believing in the project from day one and helping me navigate the unfamiliar territory along the way. Thank you to Leigh Lassiter, Kristina Horne, and everyone at TIPS Technical Publishing, Inc., for your part.

To my acquiring editor, Natalie Foreman, and the whole team at McFarland and Toplight, for agreeing to make this book a reality. Thank you for investing in this project.

To my photographer, Mike Cadotte, for being so patient and steady during those long photo shoots and coming through (as usual) with the great images that brought this book to life. Thank you for going above and beyond what was expected.

To my client and fellow ultramarathoner, Chris Hanson, for graciously agreeing to be a model and for calling me out on my diction and stuff.

To my dear friend Tam Turse for your brilliant spirit, constant encouragement, and friendship. Your insightful edits and feedback on the book were invaluable.

To Jennipher Walters and Kristen Seymour, my editors and friends at Fit Bottomed Girls, for your well-timed emails of support and assistance with editing the book. It's an honor to know you and work with you.

To my lifestyle design coach, Carl Paoli, for helping me to think clearly every step of the way. You asked all the right questions at all the right times and always reminded me to be crystal clear in thought, word, and purpose. Working with you, my friend, has been life changing. Thanks for taking a chance on me.

To my friend Quinzy Fraser for giving me a quick shot of tough love right when I needed it most. It made all the difference in how this story ended.

To my friend and colleague Sabina Grewel for allowing me the use of her Yoga Bliss Studios space to capture the photos. It's hard to imagine a more generous and kind soul than yours.

To my friends at RAD for making such incredible products. Special thanks to Joshua Hensley and his team for always making sure I have what I need.

To my lululemon family at the Westfield Montgomery Mall for all the support throughout the entire process as well as your help in selecting the right gear for the photos.

To my yoga students and clients for being my unwitting test subjects and reminding me every day why the work I do is so important through your thoughtful questions, observations, and feedback. You were (and continue to be) my biggest source of inspiration and your stories of success are what fueled me to keep writing.

To the teachers who've shared their wisdom and experience with me over the past year and challenged me to think differently—specifically Tiffany Cruikshank, Jason Crandell, Jules Mitchell, Todd Garcia, Gil Hedley, and Alexandria Crow.

To all my teachers for inspiring me to be better, with special gratitude to Susan Mondi and Jessica Apo for opening the door.

I'm so grateful for all my family, friends, and followers who have supported me since boldly leaving my corporate career to pursue this path of serving others. It's been an awesome adventure.

Foreword by Sage Rountree

Like Alison Heilig, I've been on both sides of the yoga-for-athletes combination. Yoga helped me immensely as an amateur distance runner and triathlete. The physical poses conferred strength in my core, integrity in my joints, and endurance in my muscles. The mental awareness yoga gave me helped me stay present as things got increasingly more intense in my faster and longer workouts. Best of all, yoga gave me mindful awareness that allowed me to compete at my best. Yoga supported me in a requalifying time at the Boston Marathon and kept me calm as I swam in wild seas at the 2008 World Triathlon Age-Group Championships. As an endurance sports coach and as a yoga teacher, I encourage my clients and students to incorporate yoga for its physical and mental benefits. Over the last decade, I've written several books on this intersection, including *The Athlete's Guide to Yoga*, *The Runner's Guide to Yoga*, *Everyday Yoga*, and *Lifelong Yoga*, and I've offered workshops both for athletes looking to include yoga in their training plans and for teachers interested in working with teams.

That's how I came to know Alison. A few years ago, she appeared in my workshops at the Kripalu Center for Yoga and Health in western Massachusetts, starting with my weekend workshop for athletes and continuing for an intensive for teachers who want to work with athletes. These programs run back to back, and on the afternoon between the two programs Alison and I went for a run through Lenox. Much of our conversation from this run still sticks with me. She described her running and the injuries that had plagued her—I still vividly remember exactly where we were on the route when she detailed her hip stress fracture. I heard how these injuries had led her to specialize in corrective exercises and how she included this useful work with her coaching clients and yoga students. By the end of the run, I knew Alison would be a valuable addition to the teachers' intensive, and by the end of the week, I knew I'd want Alison to return the next year

1

as my assistant. Not only did Alison's background help her contribute useful knowledge that helped her colleagues to learn, her natural sensitivity and people skills greatly enhanced everyone's experience.

As I've seen in our ongoing friendship and in Alison's interactions with her clients and her peers, her specialty is combining true durability with vulnerability: she shares her difficulties, her mistakes, and her moments of self-doubt, and every interaction with her is more human because of her honest approach. That's what you'll get from this book: the benefits of Alison's hard-earned experience combined with her belief that you can help make yourself a more durable and happy runner.

Alison's approach to making you a more durable runner is multi-pronged, so you can choose what works for you. You'll benefit from her experience as a corrective exercise specialist, as a yoga teacher, as a running coach, as a CrossFit coach, as an aficionada of self-massage techniques, and as a positive influence in the lives of her students and readers. Like any good coach, she is simultaneously playing bad cop and good cop. As I like to paraphrase the words of Peter Finley Dunne, like a good coach, she comforts the afflicted and afflicts the comfortable. She'll encourage you to push beyond your comfort level when it's helpful, to recognize the habits that don't help you. At the same time, Alison will remind you that rest is sometimes best and that you get to choose your own goals to define success for yourself.

Along the way, you will learn interesting and important information about what's happening in your body during your workouts and your daily life. Alison's presentation of anatomy is especially clear and specific to what you need to know as a runner. When you understand what's happening in your body as you train for running, you can identify where you generate imbalances in your body. Recognizing these imbalances is the first step toward fixing them, and Alison's goal in this book is to help you pinpoint the problem areas, then discern which of the many useful approaches she outlines will be the best one for you. With her help, you'll find the way to get the biggest durability payoff for your personal needs in the smallest amount of time.

Whether you are trying to achieve a personal record, conquer a new distance, overcome a history of running injuries, or simply become more centered and mentally aware, here you'll find what you need to be a more durable and happy runner.

Sage Rountree is the co-owner of Carolina Yoga Company, Hillsborough Spa and Day Retreat, and Carolina Massage Institute.

Preface

One thing is certain: I've had my fair share of running injuries. From chronic IT band issues, to a joint dislocation in my foot, to being plagued by Piriformis Syndrome, to raging shin splits, to multiple stress fractures, I've dealt with the seemingly endless frustration of running-related aches and pains. In high school and college, I'd never really considered myself to be athletic and part of what drew me to running as an adult was its apparent simplicity—you just lace up your shoes and hit the road. Turns out, it wasn't that simple at all—at least not for me. For the first nine years of my running career, I spent what seems like very little time uninjured.

With all those injuries, I naturally went through more than one period of thinking that I just wasn't built for running. Perhaps the sport didn't—and quite possibly never would—really agree with me. I envied the other runners who could run fast so fluidly and tackle high mileage with greater ease. I wondered what was so different about me and my body that I always paid for my long runs and races for days after them.

For a while, I wore the everyday aches and pains that accumulated from running like badges of honor, as symbols for the world to see of how dedicated I was to the sport. But as these things very often do, the aches and pains started to become more frequent, ultimately morphing into the occasional limp, missed days of training, and subsequent doctors' appointments. My family, friends, and colleagues began to question why I continued to do this to myself. Admittedly, I often wondered that too. Perhaps I'm just a glutton for punishment, or maybe my trademark stubbornness made it difficult for me to know when to quit. But as I befriended more and more runners, it seemed pretty normal for a runner to have something wonky going on in her body at any given moment. So I carried on.

Ultimately, it was the news of the stress fracture in my hip shortly

3

after my 30th birthday and the subsequent recovery that led me to dig deeper. As my orthopedist delivered the news, I wondered how this could have happened to me. For the first time, out loud and to another human being, I asked my orthopedist the question that had been swirling around in my head for years: "Should I stop running?"

Like many people, I assumed that because I've been running—in some form or another—since I was two years old, I knew what I was doing and my body could handle it. But what I failed to recognize is that my body had changed significantly since those days of playing in the yard. For many years, instead of running around, chasing my brother or the dog, I'd spent a number of hours sitting in classrooms at school, commuting in my car, and working at a desk job. As a result, the muscles around my hips had changed and become imbalanced. My lifestyle had created a body that was really good at sitting for long periods of time but not so great at running. In order to undo this patterning I'd unknowingly conditioned into my body, I needed to focus on building more balanced strength and stability around my hips.

After nearly a year of very limited activity as well as months of near constant pain, eventually I was given the green light to run again and I swore that I would never let myself be in this position again. I really liked and respected both my orthopedist and physical therapist, but I didn't want to have their office numbers memorized or be on a first name basis with them anymore. I didn't want to feel like I was trapped in a body that was falling apart. I wanted to feel like I had some control over how my body functioned. I wanted to feel less fragile. So I took my orthopedist's advice to do more than just run and created a new training blueprint. And with that, my concept of "durability training" was born.

After I made a great comeback from the hip fracture, there were a few other bumps in the road in the years that followed but each injury I encountered presented another opportunity for me to learn and expand on my durability training model. My struggles with IT band pain during a pair of back-to-back marathons in 2013 led me to create a comprehensive hip strength and stability program that ultimately provided long-lasting relief from pain in my knees, hips, and lower back. After stubbornly (and unwisely) running through shin splints, I ended up with a stress fracture in my shin and ultimately I learned to take better care of my lower legs. Piece by piece, injury by injury, I was building a more durable body. Before long, other runners began to seek me out to help them manage their own injuries and I realized that I was not alone.

From there, my concept of durability training really took off. I deepened my studies in anatomy, physiology, biomechanics, and corrective exercise to find ways to create better, more sustainable movement. I became a running coach and personal trainer and started working with other runners who were experiencing injury issues. I started practicing yoga and meditation regularly to build more awareness, focus, and presence. I also created and implemented a running-specific routine of targeted mobility work and strengthening exercises designed to bring my whole body back into balance—not just those areas that had been directly affected by injury. I was no longer interested in using a Band-Aid-on-a-bullet-wound approach. My goal was to be more resilient, and in order to make that a reality, I needed to think bigger picture and treat my body like it was a complete system, not just pieces that made up a whole. After a few months, I felt so confident in the work I'd done that I signed up to run my first 50K race.

While training for that first ultramarathon, for the first time in my life, I felt like running was finally agreeing with me. My running stride felt more balanced and powerful—like I was born to run. I'd become physically and mentally durable enough to withstand the rigors of high-volume training. And as I stepped up to the starting line, I felt ready. I finished feeling happy, healthy, and fully redeemed—a moment of triumph that had been (quite literally) years in the making. I'd worked so hard for so many years to overcome what seemed like a long chain of insurmountable obstacles. But in that moment, I knew that I really did have some control over what happens to me, I wasn't stuck with the hand I'd been dealt, and I could make changes that would positively alter the course of my life. It was the most empowering moment of my life.

From that point on, everything was different for me. Over the next few years, I went on to complete another five ultramarathons, many more marathons, and a number of obstacle course races—all without a single injury. In the past few years, I've started competing in CrossFit competitions as well and, now in my late 30s, I'm proud to say that my body has never been stronger or more resilient than it is right now. It's an awesome feeling to not always be waiting for the other shoe to drop, wondering if the next injury would be the one that really messes me up and keeps me from being able to not just run but to live a normal, pain-free life. Instead, I can get up every day knowing that I'm durable enough to handle whatever life throws at me. It's life changing.

As I look back now on the numerous injuries I've sustained in my running career, I can't help but feel somewhat grateful. The news that I'd fractured my hip felt like the end of the world—but it was really only the beginning. The journey to find a way to be more resilient didn't just change my relationship with this sport, it changed my entire life. Because of what I'd been through, I changed the way I treated my body. Rather than forcing it or trying to overpower or outsmart it, I began to work with it. I became a dedicated student of the body, and my desire to never be in this position again fueled a fascination with healing from the inside out. I overhauled my entire way of training to focus more on durability and resilience through understanding and compassion. Most importantly, through it all, I learned to recognize my own power to change and then truly take ownership of my role in creating a new path forward for myself—something that transcends the sport of running and permeates every aspect of my life. It doesn't feel good to feel "broken," but sometimes it's just the thing it takes to change the course of history.

That heart-breaking moment in my doctor's office was the catalyst that led me to become a running coach, a corrective exercise specialist, a yoga teacher, to leave my twelve-year career in litigation and corporate contracts, and, ultimately, to sit down and write this book. Over the years, I've worked with many people—including runners, triathletes, obstacle course racers, and CrossFit athletes—who found themselves in a similar position as I'd been in, wanting to participate more fully in life only to find themselves constantly experiencing setbacks, injury, and pain. My unique approach has helped new runners navigate the growing pains of coming into the sport and many other athletes reclaim their ability to train comfortably and consistently following chronic injury issues and traumatic accidents. I'm proud that my work has helped others improve their performance in their sport, but I'm more proud of how my durability training model has profoundly impacted my clients' performance in their lives and the way they see themselves and their capabilities. I teach and coach because I believe in human potential—yes, even yours. I believe that we all have the capacity to heal, adapt, and change. And I believe that when you finish this book, you will too.

It's because of the difficult experiences I've had that I've made it my life's work to help others feel less fragile and more empowered to take back some control over what's happening in their own bodies—not simply to chalk things up to age or some false belief that they are damaged in some unalterable way. This is my hope for every athlete and client I work with. And it's my hope for you as well. I want you to walk away from this book feeling that you can move through your life with a greater sense of confidence, knowing that you have the necessary knowledge and tools to get you on the way to becoming a more durable runner. I want you feel more resilient and capable.

But above all, I want you to believe in your own power to effect meaningful change within yourself. Because in the end, it's not just about running—it's about how you approach every aspect of your life.

You are not weak. You are not powerless. And you are not alone.

What Does It Mean to Be Durable?

Running is known to be an activity that involves injury. If you've experienced that firsthand, this book will help you become a more durable runner. Durability is the ability to withstand the inherent physical and mental stress that comes with participating in and training for sport—in your case, running. This sport is demanding. For most of us, it's what we love about it—the challenge of rising to meet those demands and the fulfillment that comes from accomplishing the things we've set out to do. So it stands to reason that we would need to prepare ourselves physically and mentally to absorb the demands of running in order to continue to participate in a meaningful and enjoyable way.

No one likes to be injured—at least no one I've ever met. However, injury is the likely result when you're unable to withstand the stresses that running places on your body and your mind. Most of the injuries that occur among runners can be traced back to the repetitive nature of the sport. In other words, most running injuries are from overuse—or, as we'll examine in this book, lack of balance.

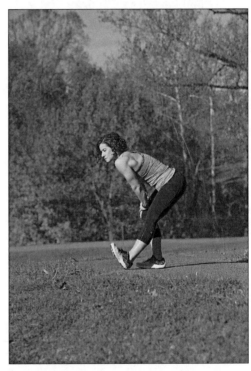

This sport is demanding. You should train to meet those demands.

If you're not durable, you can't improve. Improvement in this sport—as with any other aspect of life—comes from specific training and introducing more challenge progressively over time. Therefore, your running performance depends largely on your ability to do the work. You have to be able to continue to show up—physically and mentally—for training and hit your paces and distances. If you're hurt or even just feeling a little banged up or otherwise burnt out, you're less likely to be willing or able to give the level of effort and intensity necessary for better performance and faster race times.

Beyond the tangible benefits durability training confers for injury prevention and improved performance, many other benefits tie in. We all search for enjoyment and fulfillment when deciding to participate or continue to participate in this sport. Many of us look to the sport as a way to manage stress in other areas of our lives, or to act as the mechanism that leads us to personal growth and development. But it's hard to enjoy something that's beating you up or leaving you feeling frustrated about your lack of progress.

I've yet to meet a single runner that has stuck with the sport for any length of time that isn't getting something of value out of it. Therefore, in order to continue to reap the benefits of running, we have to be able—physically and mentally—to run. So while the concept of durability may sound incredibly simple and straightforward, it has far-reaching implications.

The Elements of Physical Durability

Physical durability refers to the resilience of the different systems and tissues in your body as well as their collective ability to work together to absorb, withstand, and bounce back from the stress placed on them as a result of training and racing. The goal of training for durability is to find a way to be able to participate physically in the sport without experiencing unnecessary wear and tear that could lead to injury or degeneration of the structures within your body.

Generally, when you learn anatomy, you learn that the muscles and other soft tissues of your body are all separate things living together under your skin. To some degree, I'll even present a bit of it that way myself in this book. While that simplification is often necessary in order to grasp what is a really complicated subject, in reality these tissues are all interconnected and dependent on each other. When someone sustains an injury that is not related to an acute trauma (such as a fall or collision), there isn't one thing you can point to that caused it. That's simply not how the body functions or dysfunctions.

Human movement is a function of the neuromusculoskeletal system—as the name suggests, it's comprised of the nervous, muscular, and skeletal systems. These three systems work together to create movement and are typically referred to as the human movement system (HMS). When looking at durability within the context of movement, then, you should consider all parts of the system—the durability of your joints, your muscles, and the connective tissues that move and support your joints as well as the ability of your nervous system to create proper muscular firing patterns and to tolerate and respond appropriately to stress.

In order for your body to be durable enough to manage the physical stress related to running, three things need to happen: (1) the support system in and around your joints needs to be balanced and stable in order to allow for proper joint alignment and function; (2) each muscle must be able to move (shorten and extend) without significant constriction; and (3) there has to be sufficient opportunity for the tissues and systems in your body to recover and adapt.

Let's explore these components individually.

Proper Joint Function and Support

When you look at an illustration or a model of the human skeleton, it appears as though there is a space between the bones of the major joints. For example, when you look at an image of a hip joint, it appears as though the knob at the top of the thighbone sits in the hip socket with a little room to spare. In reality, though, there is no space there. That void you see is actually filled with all sorts of interesting and important stuff.

So let's break the hip joint down into its layers. First, both the knobby end of your thighbone and the hip socket itself are lined with a thin layer of cartilage that provides a layer of protection for the bones. In addition to the cartilaginous lining, you have a thicker, cushiony pad of fibrous cartilage, called the labrum, that lines the rim of your hip socket and acts as a rubber gasket to keep your thighbone in the socket. The next layer is the joint capsule, which seals everything in like a Ziploc bag. Over all those structures are ligaments that reinforce the joint capsule and tie your bones together so things don't move around too much in there. Then you have some bursa, strategically placed sacs of fluid that provide cushioning between surfaces and secrete lubrication so the joint can move well without a bunch of friction.

These structures inside the joint provide some passive stability, which means they stabilize the joint in a way that you don't and can't actively control. But these structures afford only a small amount of the joint stabilization properties you need in order to keep your joints healthy and mobile for life. Fortunately for you, over the top of these delicate structures are sophisticated communities of muscles and tendons designed to position things precisely inside the allotted joint space—providing more active stabilization for your joints through muscular tone and engagement. Each muscle within the community has a specific job to do—whether that be moving, stabilizing, or a little of both. When the joint is balanced and working smoothly, each muscle does its part to ensure that the constituent parts fit together nicely and can move around without bumping and grinding into things they shouldn't be (such as the cartilage, labrum or meniscus, and bursa).

When the community is working well, the system works well. If one muscle starts pulling more than another or if any of them stops doing their job, the joint doesn't align well and continued movement can result in things pressing into and irritating other things inside the joint. In addition, when the forces pulling on the joint become unbalanced, the underlying ligaments can get strained from having to do more of the stabilization work.

The goal, then, is to build a functioning community of muscles that is supportive enough to properly stabilize your joints. Not only is it more efficient in terms of movement, it's also how you limit the amount of potentially irreversible wear and tear that occurs inside your joints. Since the protective cartilage that lines your bones doesn't contain nerves, you might not feel that there's an issue in there until you wear through this critical protective layer and find yourself with bones that are grinding into each other with every step you take. Ouch.

KEY POINT: *The Movers and the Stabilizers*

There are muscles in your body that are probably fairly familiar to you even if you're not particularly interested in anatomy. There are also many muscles that are far less familiar but often are more critical to consider when it comes to injury prevention. Anatomy books are designed to provide clarity and simplify the arrangement of muscles by showing each muscle separately and with clearly delineated and specific functions. While that is essential for learning, in reality, bodies are far more complicated than that. You are made up of many layers of muscle, and each muscle does more than one thing.

Throughout this book, I'll be classifying muscles based on their primary functions as movers or stabilizers. Generally speaking, the bigger, easier-to-recognize muscles (like your quads and lats) are the more superficial mover muscles and the smaller, less familiar ones (like your gluteus medius and serratus anterior) are the deeper layers of muscles that stabilize your joints.

This distinction is made for the sake of simplicity; many muscles do a little of both to some degree. Keep sight of the bigger picture: in order for a joint to move efficiently with minimal wear and tear to the underlying joint structures (such as the capsule, cartilage, labrum or meniscus, etc.), the muscles that move and position the bones within the joint need to work together as a community. Movers and stabilizers unite!

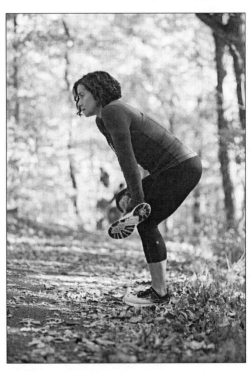

Durability training is about restoring a global sense of balance to the runner.

Proper Tissue Quality and Function

In addition to supporting and stabilizing your joints so that the passive joint structures are not being pressed against and irritated, your muscles must be capable of moving your bones so you can get around. Most of us are familiar with the idea of muscle contraction, but this is really only part of the equation.

First, your muscles need to be excitable, meaning that they respond appropriately when your nervous system tells them to do something. Much of this is initially learned during early childhood development—as you start to explore the world, your brain is wiring up your movement patterns and learning to coordinate movement by activating specific muscle fibers. If you've ever tried some new activity and felt really clumsy with it at first but got better at it after a few repetitions, you've experienced your nervous system figuring out how to create a new, coordinated movement. Once your nervous system figures out where to send the message, your muscles need to be able to respond to it.

Obviously, your muscles also need to be able to contract, or shorten, when stimulated. This is how bones move through space. Equally important, though, is your muscles' ability to stop contracting and instead release so that the fibers can be stretched enough to allow for other surrounding muscles to contract and do their jobs. Movement occurs through an oppositional lever system. Consider your traditional biceps curl—in order to curl the weight to your shoulder, your biceps contract to bend your elbow. At the same time, the muscle fibers in your triceps have to release enough to let your biceps shorten. It's like a very civilized tug-of-war match. If all goes well, the joint can move efficiently and smoothly through its full range of motion.

Skeletal muscles are the most adaptive tissues in your body—the more you use them, they better they function. When you contract your muscles, blood flows in to keep them properly oxygenated. Muscles are also amazingly resilient. When a muscle is stressed beyond its current capability, the individual fibers that make up the muscle are damaged. Then, as you rest the muscle, your immune system activates special cells that go in there, multiply, and fuse themselves to the damaged muscle fibers. These newly repaired fibers are stronger and more resilient than the old ones—think of it as your muscles' way of laying down an insurance policy against future damage just in case you ever decide to stress it out like that again. But since muscles are so frequently and relatively easily damaged, you really don't want your muscles connecting straight to your bones and having the responsibility of pulling on them. So instead, you have tendons.

Tendons are tough connective tissues that attach your muscles to your bones. They are capable of withstanding more tension and force than your muscles so they can pull on your bones without tearing. Tendons—like ligaments—are meant to be strong and relatively inflexible; in fact, their proper function depends on it. They have to have enough give to absorb force and allow things to move around a little while also maintaining a firm boundary for how far things can go. If a tendon is subjected to chronic tension—whether that be from repetitive movements or muscular tightness—there is potential for it to become inflamed, which is painful and can interfere with your ability to move well.

Movement constriction can also result from dehydration and adhesions in your fascia. Fascia is connective tissue that not only forms a wrapper around your muscles but also runs through them. Fascia encases and connects every tissue in your body in one long, uninterrupted, continuous network. Healthy fascia has a certain balance of collagen fibers for strength, elastin fibers for elasticity, and a gel-like substance that helps lubricate the tissues so that the layers of tissue glide over each other easily as you move. Fascial dehydration occurs when the gel-like substance thickens, which creates friction in areas where the tissues should otherwise be able to glide fluidly over each other. Adhesions are an over-accumulation of collagen fibers that can cause the layers of tissue to become stuck to each other like Velcro, causing tissues to pull on other surrounding tissues during movement. Both of these scenarios can create an uncomfortable feeling of tightness in your body and enough tissue restriction to decrease your mobility.

You need your muscles, tendons, and fascia all to be happy, healthy, and fully functional so that your joints are free to move through their entire range of motion to keep you running well. Constriction in any of these tissues can negatively affect the whole community (including the joint itself), creating potential for overuse of certain tissues, compensation by other tissues, and ultimately joint pain, dysfunction, and degeneration.

Adequate Recovery and Restoration

Your nervous system consists of your brain and spinal cord (the central nervous system) as well as all the other nerves that branch off of your spinal cord and run through your entire body (the peripheral nervous system). The functions of your peripheral nervous system can be divided into two buckets: the stuff you control voluntarily or consciously (the somatic nervous system) and the stuff that happens automatically (the autonomic nervous system).

Within the autonomic nervous system, there are the two systems that control your physiological responses to the world around you—they are the sympathetic and parasympathetic nervous systems. The sympathetic nervous system governs the fight/flight/freeze responses in your body, and it is triggered any time you're in danger or perceive a threat. Activation of this system triggers a chain reaction of events in your body, releasing chemicals that are designed to temporarily divert energy away from nonessential organ functions—such as digestion and some immune functions—so that your body can use that energy to keep you alive by increasing your heart rate to fully prime and oxygenate your muscles, releasing stored energy into your bloodstream, heightening your senses, and increasing your lungs' ability to take in oxygen. This is all incredibly helpful when you're in legitimate fear for your life. Evolutionarily, this ability has served us well.

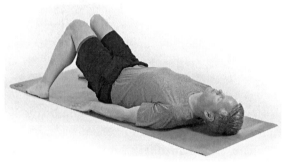

Sometimes less really is more.

The problem is that instead of that system being activated only in case of life-threatening emergencies and lasting only for a short while, you can get stuck in this mode. Typically, these fight/flight/freeze chemicals are meant to dissipate as your body breaks them down, so you can return to normal functions and not constantly feel like you're about to have to run for your life. However, the stresses of dealing with daily life and traumatic events can lead to a nearly constant low-grade stream of chemicals dripping into your system. And as that becomes more and more normal, you might not even register it as an issue. Instead, you might just feel "off" or report feeling a little anxious.

Remember that this is meant to be a temporary response system, not the way you live your life. If the response is not interrupted and reset periodically, bad things start to happen. The systems your nervous system shut down are really important to your overall health, and they aren't meant to be shut down for long. Your body isn't meant to stew in the stress chemicals released by your nervous system.

The way you reset the system and keep your sympathetic nervous system from chronically hijacking the normal and necessary functions of your body is by tapping into parasympathetic mode. Your parasympathetic nervous system is responsible for the "rest and digest" functions of your body, otherwise known as the relaxation response—but there's way more to this response than just being "chill." When your parasympathetic nervous system is in charge, important tasks get done. Your organs return to their normal relaxed states: you digest food, your heart does its thing in a relaxed and efficient way, your immune system goes to work keeping you healthy, your metabolism normalizes, and even your breathing requires less effort.

This downtime is when many critical functions occur that make it possible for you to run well and recover fully. For example, your food is broken down into parts that can be used by your body for energy and tissue repair, normal sleep patterns resume, and your muscles can release tension and rebuild. The challenge is remembering (and then taking the time) to consciously flip the switch. Recovery is not guaranteed, friends—you have a role to play here. Don't worry, though: I have tons of ideas to share with you in the pages that follow.

The Elements of Mental Durability

Mental durability is the resilience of your mind and refers to its ability to withstand the stress caused by the rigors of training and racing without leading to burnout or mental fatigue. This has been an overlooked and undervalued aspect of training. Intuitively, we know that training can certainly take a toll on us physically—why wouldn't it also have the potential to do so mentally? We should take steps to prepare for and counter this toll.

Too often, runners assume that mental toughness is something you're born with—a quality you either have or you don't. But mental durability and toughness are skills, and just like every other skill you want to acquire in life, you have to develop them through practice.

There are five key components of mental durability: presence, focus, grit, adaptability, and growth mindedness. When these skills are trained and developed well, you are better equipped to define success for yourself, read your own gauge, dig deep and push through when necessary, pivot and find a new path forward when things don't go your way, and handle pressure as well as deal with failures and setbacks.

All of the above take time and practice to develop. You have to train your brain for running the way you train your body. Through repetition and reinforcement, you can develop your ability to recognize what you're working with today, to stay focused in the face of distraction, to bounce back from bad training runs, to stay on track when motivation is nowhere to be found, and to carry on after a setback. But most importantly, as the intensity of your training or daily stress levels increase, you have to learn how to flip the switch and let your mind recover the same way you let your body recover. You cannot expect that continued overloading of the system will elicit good results.

Almost every runner has had a mental injury related to the sport at some point. Mental injuries are common in runners because the mental aspect of training in the general population is still so overlooked. Mental injuries can also be the hardest to put your finger on in identifying the cause and the remedy. When left unresolved, burnout can lead people to reluctantly leave the sport that once brought them so much joy and fulfillment. When you proactively include mental durability training, it becomes much easier to prevent both mental and physical injuries. Additionally, you won't just improve your mindset when it comes to running, you'll increase your tolerance for dealing with challenges and setbacks in every area of your life. You'll be a more durable runner.

It All Boils Down to Balance

By now you should be noticing a theme: the goal is balance. There needs to be balance around your joints to keep them aligned and moving well, balance within the tissues themselves in their ability to perform their functions well, and balance between challenge and rest. Most injuries runners experience are linked to an imbalance in one or more of these areas. When things are not in balance, parts of the system start to break down faster than they can be repaired.

That's not to say that injuries mean you've failed in some way. Arguably, the more you play with your edge in order to see how good you really can be in this sport, the further from balance you need to be, and injury could very well be inevitable as a result. This book will provide you with information to understand how you might have ended up injured or burnt out—and more importantly, it provides a roadmap for how you might get yourself out of that place and move forward.

While injury prevention is the goal of this book, injuries are simply a form of feedback—often very valuable feedback. Time and time again, runners have chosen to take the feedback injury provides them and use it to come back stronger, more aware, and more compassionate. My own story is full of times when I can look back and say that there have been many lessons in the healing process.

But there are things you can and should do to help minimize your chances of getting hurt, especially if you are dealing with chronic injuries or simply looking to continue enjoying the sport and limit the amount of interruption injury causes in your training and in your life. It is possible to train in a way that pushes your limits enough to improve your race times and performance without significantly increasing your injury risk—you just have to do it in a balanced way. This book is here to help you do just that.

The Causes of Imbalance

There are many reasons why imbalance might occur in runners. In order to figure out what's happening with you specifically, you have to engage in the process of self-study and increase your awareness of yourself and your habits. Only you can really figure it out. Once you've finished this book, you'll be in a position to understand what might be contributing to any issues you're experiencing and I hope that you'll share that information with your healthcare providers, coaches, and physical therapists so you can continue to correct those imbalances. Here are three of the most common sources of imbalance I see in runners.

Repetitive Stress

Running is a repetitive motion sport—in other words, you do the same thing over and over. That isn't a bad thing. Remember that your body is highly adaptable. The problem is when all that repetitive motion isn't balanced out by spending time in other positions and when it isn't followed by the appropriate amount of rest.

As we'll explore in the chapters that follow, each joint is capable of doing multiple actions that move the bones in more than one direction. Running, however, involves repetitive movements that disproportionately emphasize one joint action over others. Absent appropriate intervention and regular exposure to other movements, the balance within the communities of muscles around those joints can be disrupted.

Think of overuse not as an indicator that you've used a part of your body too much and exceeded its reasonable lifespan, but consider usage in terms of proportionality. Your body was meant to move, and it functions better when moved frequently. As you'll see in the next chapter, most of the cells in your body are constantly turning over and being replaced with new cells. So the concept that you've gotten injured because you've somehow exceeded the recommended usage hours for your body is absurd.

No, overuse is a relative term—meaning you've used one part of your body out of proportion with the other parts or you've worked it more than you've rested it. In other words, there is a lack of balance. It could be that you've used it so much that it becomes dominant and starts compensating for weaker muscles within the community. You could have used it so much that it's fatigued and simply trying to tell you to give it a break. You could have used it so much that tension has built up in the muscles or tendons from insufficient or poor rest quality. It could mean that you've spent more time shortening the muscle than extending it. Or you could have just been neglecting the other muscles in the community in favor of using the same muscle over and over in the same way. Whatever the cause, something has become unbalanced.

In order to get better at running, you have to run—that is inescapable. But running alone is not enough to stay healthy. Running can condition your heart and running muscles well, but what about the remaining muscles? How is doing the same thing over and over again going to lead you closer to balance? It's not. You have to do other things. You have to be mindful of how much time you spend conditioning your muscles to contract in the very specific way they move while you're running versus the amount of time you spend releasing your running muscles and contracting the other muscles within that community. Otherwise, things start to get irritated, and that's when you start to see the inflammation or "-itis" injuries that tend to be so common among runners.

Postural Patterns and Habits

There is often this belief among people that since running is something that most of us have been doing since we were very young we should all be naturally good at it. Well, that was definitely not my experience, and it's not the experience of most people who came to the sport later in life. There are several reasons for that.

First and foremost, a lot has changed in your body since you were a kid. Your body, the awesomely adaptive structure that it is, has modeled itself along the lines of the things you do most often—a subject we'll dive deeper into in the next chapter. For many of us, that means our bodies have adapted to a lot of time spent sitting, which, like the repetitive motion of running, can lead to some overspecialization in the tissues and ultimately imbalance in the communities of muscles around your joints. Many of the injuries I see in new runners or those who are returning to the sport after some time away are related to this phenomenon—meaning that they try to take their "sitting body" out for a run. The tissues in your body might put up with that for a short while and over short distances, but ultimately they will start to complain.

This can be problematic for many reasons. Let's consider the hip joint. Sitting involves passive hip flexion—meaning that if you spend your day at a desk like most people, the angle of your hip joint from torso to

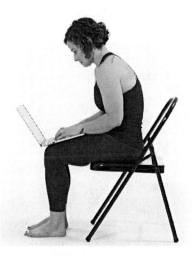

Poor postural habits can change the length and function of your soft tissues over time.

thigh is about 90 degrees. Because your thighs are resting on a seat, this hip flexion is passive, meaning that the muscles that flex your hip (your hip flexors) are shortened but not contracted. And your hips remain in that position for large parts of the day. The result is that the front of your hips over time can become tight and weak. Running requires a different set-up—at least if you want to run comfortably. To run well, you need strong hip flexors that also lengthen to allow for your glutes and hamstrings to extend your leg behind you and propel you forward powerfully.

These patterns don't just show up in the hips—the way you position your lower back as well as your tendency to slouch and round your shoulders can also create inefficiencies in your running stride and your breathing as well as an imbalance that could ultimately result in pain or injuries in your back, shoulders, and neck.

While running might seem like a simple sport, newer runners (as well as those returning to the sport) don't always get that it's usually not as simple as one foot in front of the other. You have to train your tissues to deal with this new type of stress. Seasoned runners don't get off easy here, either. You need to be mindful of the powerful role that lifestyle plays in the way your tissues work (or don't work) together. Just one day spent sitting more than usual can have a major impact on how your evening run feels. String enough of those days together and it can start to feel like running is taking a toll on you.

Sympathetic Dominance

Many people come to the sport fairly casually. They do it because it's fun to run with their friends a couple of days a week, and soon they sign up for a local race. Usually, then they begin to enjoy the process of training for a race, as they see the incremental gains adding up. At some point, it occurs to each of us that if running three days per week helps us improve so much, then running six or seven must exponentially increase those gains. That, my friends, is a trap.

Newer runners aren't the only ones who experience this. As we saw earlier in this chapter, many of us live in a fairly constant state of sympathetic nervous system activity—it might be low-grade or it might be more extreme depending on your lifestyle and other factors—and that has become the norm. When you are in fight/flight/freeze mode, not only are you limiting your body's ability to recover, you are altering your decision-making abilities.

Eventually, it seems we all end up falling for thinking that in order to be better, we have to do more. But often, the opposite is true. I've seen many runners create ambitious training plans with intense, quality-effort runs, cross-training activities, and heated power yoga classes, thinking that this offers them a well-rounded approach to physical training. Instead, they find themselves even further from where they want to be. Then, following the introduction of a smart and balanced training plan, they realize that less really can be more.

I tell my clients that every training week should have a flow to it. Some days are hard effort and high intensity and others will be light effort and low intensity. That balanced flow must be maintained. Otherwise, you run the risk of having every day be a medium-effort and medium-intensity day because you aren't physically or mentally capable of high-intensity output on the hard-effort days as a result of overdoing it on the days that were intended to be light and easy. If you always train at medium intensity, your results will always be lukewarm, and the likelihood of burnout and injury increases. Sadly, however, this is very common. It's the result of people trying to do more when they really need to do less.

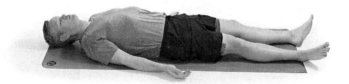

Savasana, or Corpse Pose, offers a chance to do
nothing so that your body has time to catch up.

The bottom line is this: you cannot let yourself get stuck in the fight/flight/freeze mode. It doesn't matter if the trigger is your training or other things in your life; the slow and steady stream of stress hormones adds up and compromises the functionality of the whole system. Even if you feel like you're getting enough time away from running, that doesn't mean that your body is recovering. You have to take rest preemptively as well as learn to recognize when it's time to reboot the system. Otherwise, you fall into the same old trap of thinking that more is more.

Creating Durability

Now that you understand the concept of durability, let's talk about how to get you there—and that's where the rest of this book comes in. Creating durability is really just a fancy way of saying "restoring balance." We know that running is a repetitive motion sport. We know that postural habits add up over time. We know that life has a way of limiting the amount of time we spend in relaxation mode. Combined, these factors can set you up for potential imbalance if you don't proactively seek ways to restore some balance to the way you move and the systems that support you.

Your body functions best when things are in balance and you have the ability to help restore that balance. If it took you years to get to where you are now, it will take time to undo those patterns, but small changes to the things you do every day can have a massive impact over time. My goal isn't to pile on to your to-do list, it's to give you information that allows you to implement some new daily practices that are simple and fit your life—because if you're not doing the work, it can't help you.

It all begins with awareness. If you want your body to continue to support you and the activities that bring you joy for the rest of your life, you'd better spend some time getting to know it. So the first step is investing a bit of your time getting to know yourself better so you can see where things are not balanced. It requires looking at your postural habits as well as making notes of your strengths and weaknesses. Then, once you know what you're working with, you can decide what needs to change in order to create a better balance for yourself and your body. This step provides you with your action items for moving forward. Finally, you have to practice taking those steps. This could mean developing a daily movement practice at home using the work I present in this book or changing your postural habits or taking more time in relaxation mode. Ideally, it's some combination of all of the above.

If you want to change something about what's happening in your body, you have to change your habits—the stuff you do repeatedly. You cannot keep doing the same things you're doing and expect different results. Let's explore how change occurs.

Physical Adaptation

Your body is constantly changing. Throughout your lifetime, the cells and fibers of your body are being turned over according to a specific timeline and being replaced with new cells and fibers that are specifically adapted to the tasks, habits, patterns, and positions that you most frequently experience and perform. This is your body's way of becoming more efficient. The more you're exposed to something, the better you become at handling it. For example, the first time you do a workout, it's challenging and you'll probably feel sore the next day. Then the next time you do that same workout, it's not so bad.

I believe that this is one of the greatest qualities that our bodies possess—their adaptability. Much of it goes unnoticed. Often we look at our bodies and the way that they've adapted to life as a dysfunction—but it's the opposite that's true. Typically, your body adapts in an attempt to make you more functional within the context of the environment that you're frequently subjected to. You might not like the result of it and it might make doing other things that you do less frequently more challenging and potentially injurious, but your body is doing the best it can.

As frustrating as it may be when your body adapts to your lifestyle and treatment of it in a way that you don't find favorable, it really is an incredible process. The body finds a way to carry on, and it does so quickly and gracefully. The things that anatomy books might label as dysfunction are actually very often small miracles of adaptation—your body's intelligence applied to forge greater strength and resilience in response to the stresses and demands that are being placed on it.

Physical adaptation is not a haphazard thing, nor is it a fluke—it happens for a reason, in response to something that you're doing a lot of. If you're unhappy with where you've ended up, you should consider changing what you're doing and the frequency with which you do it. Many runners who've experienced injury issues speak about their bodies as if their bodies are broken or turning against them. It's heartbreaking to hear, especially because I've been there too.

I hope to reframe the way you think about adaptation, to build a greater understanding of the process. With understanding comes compassion, and the best and most productive relationships are built on a foundation of compassion. Once you understand the mechanisms that create adaptation, you have the power to change the things you're doing in order to affect the way your body is adapting. Understanding is the key to changing course and to realizing that not everything is out of your control. Once you understand how the system works, you can start working with the system rather than against it—and ultimately you'll find that what's happening in your body is not as mysterious as you might have once thought.

There are no quick fixes or magic beans. You get out of your body exactly what you put into it. If you give your body appropriate and progressive amounts of challenge, adequate quality recovery, proper tissue maintenance work, periodic nervous system resets, solid mindset awareness practice, plenty of sleep, and balanced nutrition, I bet things will start to improve quickly and dramatically. It's not rocket science. The basic stuff works.

KEY POINT: *Movement Compensations—Good or Bad?*

Every part of your body has a specific job to do, and your body operates best when everything is working well and cooperating. Things don't always happen that way in reality, but your body will still find a way to carry on as best it can. Movement compensations are one such way.

Movement compensation is a term that has developed a negative connotation in the fitness industry. It's often talked about as though it's some sort of dysfunction in the way your body moves. But I believe this severely underestimates what bodies are capable of.

In my work, I find that most movement compensations are simply adaptations that the body moves toward as a result of something else—such as chronic pain, tension, restriction, trauma, or instability. This is a testament to how smart your body really is. There are things happening in your body that don't register on the intellectual level. Your body is constantly collecting internal information about joint positions and tissue tension all day, every day in order to keep you safe. If your body finds an issue that it can't fix directly, or if you were to ignore its messages long enough, it will find a way to circumvent it to keep you functioning as best it can. It's amazing how adaptable we are!

While movement compensations are something that need to be addressed in situations where they are negatively affecting joint alignment and function, causing pain or damage, or otherwise creating inefficiencies in the way you move, we need to stop being so angry about them when they happen. We take for granted so much when it comes to our bodies. We could—and some of us do—spend years imposing our will on them, neglecting their needs, ignoring the whispers and warning signs they send to us and yet still, somehow, in spite of it all, behind the scenes your body is constantly remodeling itself in a way that perfectly suits where you are in your life—for better or worse.

Changing Course

When you were first born, you had very few skills—pretty much only the instinctual stuff. You came with a certain amount of hardwiring, and that's about it. Fortunately, your instincts had you primed and hardwired to learn, and that was your only job for the first few years of your life. As time went on, your body started to adapt to the world around you. Your vision got clearer. You learned to coordinate your fingers in order to grab things and try to stick them in your mouth before your parents could stop you. Then you learned to crawl and eventually walk. This was only the beginning of a lifetime of learning and adapting.

But at a certain point, things change. Instead of craving and actively seeking things that make you grow and adapt, you start to fear and avoid those things. You give up some growth in order to find stability within your own personal comfort zone. As a baby, you could not have cared less about failing and making a fool of yourself, and you really had no other choice—adapting was just what you did. As an adult, it's a bit harder. Instead of adapting to new things, you've adapted to the norm, the things you do over and over. You stop changing so much and instead just deepen the grooves of routine, comfort, and habit. But you never stopped being capable of learning and growing; it's just more challenging, mentally and emotionally, when you're older and more firmly stuck in your ways.

Many people have this idea that they should have mastered how to use their own body after a few decades. But that's the error in thinking. Your body did master life, exactly the life you asked it to adapt to—but that doesn't come without risks.

You're still capable of change, and that's the crux of this book. If what you've been doing has been working for you, then by all means keep it up if that makes you happy. But if you've picked up this book, odds are something isn't working for you as well as it could be and it's time to give your body something new to adapt to in order to spark change.

The Science of Change

In order to work with your body to create positive and desirable changes to the way it moves and functions, you have to first take into consideration how your body responds and adapts to physical activity and stress over time. When you encounter a new or different type of challenge that exceeds your current capacity, it's stressful. This stress is the catalyst for change and adaptation. If you're never challenged and stressed, you and your capacity remain the same. Obviously, there is a thoughtful and intelligent way to apply this knowledge—this is the field of exercise physiology.

The first principle of exercise physiology is overloading. In order for you to improve, you have to give your body a reason to adapt by demanding a little more from it. Your body is designed to increase its capacity in response to new and different challenges. Doing things that you've already mastered won't make you better.

The second principle is one of specificity. If you want to change a habit or the way your body moves and functions, you have to train it in a way that is specific to what you hope to accomplish. For example, if you want to be able to run long distances, you won't get there by going to the gym and trying to bench press your body weight—you have to actually train to run long distances. The system you challenge and stress is the system that improves.

Think about how you currently challenge your body every day. Some of that stress is intentional, like training your body for more endurance and faster pace times. Some of that stress occurs based on the demands you place on your body as part of your lifestyle—like sitting at a desk, typing on a keyboard, or staring at mobile devices. You get better at the specific things you practice most often. What do you practice most often? What are you teaching your body to get really good at?

The third principle relates to the concept of progression. If you want to continue to improve, you have to gradually and systematically increase the challenge over time. In other words, if you want to run a marathon, you don't just go out and try to run the full 26.2 miles tomorrow. Instead, you progressively build your mileage over time with periods of reduced mileage every few weeks to allow your body to adapt to the increased physical demand. There are many different dials you can use to create change through progressive overload—intensity (how hard you run), duration (how long you run), and frequency (how often you run), for instance.

The fourth principle is the law of diminishing returns, which boils down to the idea that more is not necessarily better. The better you get at something, the more efficient your body becomes, and the less change you'll see. Most of us see the most improvement in running in our first year or two. Then we start to hit plateaus where, even though our training investments are consistent (or even higher), we don't improve as much or as quickly as we used to. When that happens, you might feel the urge to invest more by upping your mileage—but that might actually have the opposite effect. This is when we need to learn to train smarter, not harder.

The fifth principle is recovery. The more you increase the demands, the more important recovery becomes. Constantly overloading yourself without adequate time to recover leads to breakdown. Adaptation doesn't happen during the workout itself—this is the application of stress. The adaptation actually occurs when you're recovering—as you rest, your body repairs and rebuilds itself to be stronger.

The sixth principle is reversibility. Since your body adapts to the demands placed on it, when you stop demanding that it rise to a specific challenge, the gains will be lost. Basically, it's a matter of use it or lose it. And while this might, at first glance, seem like a bad thing, think of it this way: if you're dealing with injuries or discomfort and it's a result of something specific that you're doing in terms of posture or movement but you stop doing that thing, your body can readjust. All adaptations are reversible.

As a runner, these concepts are probably not foreign to you. These are the essential underlying principles of any smart physical training plan—the science behind how to change and improve your capabilities within any sport. But what we don't often think about is how these principles apply not just to our run training but also to how our bodies adapt to postural patterns and repetitive movements in our daily lives.

We know that we can use our knowledge of the adaptation process to incrementally improve running performance. Can we use this same knowledge to change habits and increase durability at the same time? I think we can.

Remember that your body is constantly changing and evolving. The question becomes what are you doing every day to ensure that the remodeling of tissues in your body occurs in a way that allows you to get better and continue to train? Are you playing a conscious and intentional role in that remodeling process or are you just crossing your fingers and hoping for the best?

How to Become More Durable

As you've seen, there's a lot that goes into being durable. But the great thing is that we all started out pretty balanced in the beginning and somewhere along the way we got really specialized and moved toward imbalance. Now you just have to get back to balance, and this book will give you the tools to do that.

I believe in a three-pronged approach. Why? Because we are complicated beings. The human movement system involves multiple parts—the nervous, muscular, and skeletal systems—that all work together. Therefore, your training to condition your own movement and functionality should too. The training protocol outlined in this book involves corrective exercise for joint mobility and muscular strength and balance, myofascial release to improve soft tissue quality and function, and yoga for self-awareness and focus.

Let's talk about how these three modalities work together to help facilitate that process.

Corrective Exercise

Corrective exercise, as defined by the National Academy of Sports Medicine (NASM), is a "systematic process of identifying a neuromusculoskeletal dysfunction, developing a plan of action, and implementing an integrated corrective strategy."* In other words, you're looking for things that aren't working as well as you'd like, coming up with a plan for how to change that, and then doing new things that help bring you back into balance. Each chapter of this book contains two focus areas for corrective work—mobility and strength/activation exercises.

Since most of us tend to spend a lot of time in the same position for most of the day, your body needs to spend some time in other positions in order to help preserve your body's ability to go there safely. The mobility work in this book involves positioning and moving your major joints into different positions to help maintain their full functional range of motion (FROM). FROM is a term used to describe the agreed-upon amounts that a joint should be able to move in all directions in order to for you to do the things that humans need to do, like crouching, reaching, crawling, carrying things, leaning, etc. Because we're talking more in terms of joint range of motion rather than soft tissue flexibility, not all of the mobility work in this book will feel like a stretch.

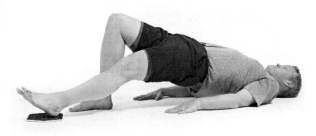

Corrective exercises create balance between strength and mobility.

The mobility work is less about increasing flexibility through stretching and more about trying to preserve the capacity of your joints and muscles to do other things. Rather than trying to aggressively pull on or "lengthen" your muscles, you'll simply put your body in a different shape for a little while so that it maintains its comfort level with that particular position. It's just a friendly little reminder to your body.

That's not to say that you won't experience a change to range of motion. If your body often feels "tight," you certainly might start to notice the feeling of being more flexible as your muscular and nervous systems feel more comfortable with your joints being in different positions again. But it's simply not necessary to wrench yourself into deeper and deeper

---

*Clark, M., Lucett, S., & Sutton, B. G. (2014). *NASM Essentials of Corrective Exercise Training* (1st ed. rev.). Burlington, MA: Jones & Bartlett Learning.

stretches to accomplish that—it might even be counterproductive as a certain amount of stiffness and tension are necessary in order to properly stabilize your joints. Save the hard efforts for your training runs.

The strength and activation exercises in this book are designed to help you see where certain muscles might not be supporting you as well as they could be. You'll do work that specifically explores each part of the community of muscles as well as some exercises that teach the entire community to work better together so that you're building strength in a way that's functional, cohesive, and integrated to better support your joints and your running form.

First and foremost, as NASM's definition suggests, the corrective exercise protocol and strategies laid out in this book are designed to help you recognize imbalances in your own body that may be contributing to movement dysfunctions or injuries. Again, awareness is key. As you work with the mobility and activation techniques, you'll notice that certain things feel comfortable and familiar to you and you'll struggle with others. The stuff you struggle with is where the magic is—anything you're not currently great at represents potential for improvement. These challenging movements are not just "testers" to see where you are, they're also the roadmap to improvement. Know that anything you find difficult or more challenging now is going to help you get better and feel better by moving you closer to balance.

After you've done the initial work of trying the things outlined in this book, you'll have a pretty clear picture of where to focus your efforts based on where you feel the most tension and what you struggle with the most. From there, the game plan is set—you'll continue to work on those areas with the goal of developing more balanced and functional range of motion in your joints, greater ease in tight, overactive tissues, greater activation and strength in underutilized muscles, and, ultimately, improved cooperation within each community of muscles.

KEY POINT: *How Much Flexibility Do Runners Need?*

When runners approach me about yoga and corrective exercise, nine times out of 10 they complain about not being able to touch their toes. For some reason, runners have gotten stuck on the thought that this is somehow a requirement of being able to run or function as a human in life—but it's really not. In my experience, athletes who naturally have very flexible hamstrings (the kind that allows a person to easily touch their toes) also have more difficulty creating enough activation and contraction in their hamstrings to properly power their running stride. More is not always better.

First, whether or not you are able to touch your toes comfortably depends on a number of factors, not just flexibility. Some of these factors might be under your control and can ultimately change through practice and training. Other factors are nonnegotiable, like bone shape or joint depth and angles. Nothing short of surgery to alter the shape of your bones will change these things. But this is not a bad thing either—as you'll learn, some structural limitations built into your body are there for good reason.

But second, and more importantly, in order to participate in the sport of running, you need enough flexibility to tie your shoes. Touching your toes with straight legs from a standing or seated position is not a prerequisite for the sport. You just need to have tissues that are flexible enough to allow your joints to move through a range of motion that creates an effective running stride. That's it.

Is wanting to touch your toes bad? No. But we would all do better

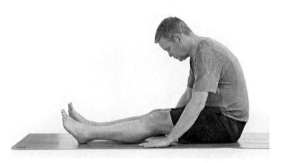

A common seated hamstring stretch.

to remind ourselves that more for the sake of more is not always better. Periodically, revisit what your intentions are. If your goal is to touch your toes, know why that matters to you. Ask yourself what specifically you are trying to gain by increasing your flexibility and whether more flexibility is truly the best method to help you make those gains for yourself. If you're desperately striving to touch your toes because you think it will make you a better runner, know that it probably won't but there are many other things that will, like building strength, moving your joints in new ways, and improving circulation to your muscles and connective tissues—all things that are covered at length in this book.

Prioritizing flexibility over other aspects of efficient movement is not an effective strategy for injury prevention. It is also not necessarily going to improve your running performance. In fact, in some athletes it can have the opposite effect since a certain amount of responsiveness and springiness is required to maintain the efficiency of your running stride. I've known many runners who can comfortably fold themselves in half who struggle with chronic hip and leg injuries and I've known plenty of runners who can barely touch their upper shins but are healthy, happy, and fast. Instead of seeking more flexibility, let's focus on achieving greater functionality.

Myofascial Release

As a runner, you spend a lot of time devoted to strengthening and conditioning your muscles for running. The muscles that move you through the miles are probably pretty familiar to you as are the concepts of muscular contraction and stretching. However, with all this emphasis on muscular conditioning, it's easy to lose sight of the fact that it's not just about your muscles—many structures and systems in your body that support your muscles also need to be properly maintained and cared for.

In the end, your muscles are really only as good as the structures that attach to them and the systems that maintain them. Neglecting this part of your anatomy makes it more challenging to get the gains you're working for in your training. As we touched on briefly in the previous chapter, fascia is a continuous web of connective tissue that wraps around, runs through, and supports every muscle and organ in your body. The cumulative effects of your posture and the repetitive motions of life and physical activity can result in tension, achiness, and restriction in this tissue that may not be improved by simply stretching your muscles.

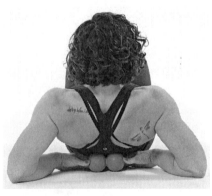

Self-myofascial release is TLC, not torture, for your tissues.

Myofascial release is a really effective way to help your body help you. Myofascial release is a catchall term that describes any technique used to manipulate your muscles and/or fascia.

Some of the most familiar forms of myofascial release are trigger point therapy, massage, acupuncture, and cupping—all of which require the assistance of a trained professional for administration. However, it is possible to perform myofascial release work on yourself—a technique called self-myofascial release (SMR). This is the technique that you'll find in this book.

In each chapter, you'll learn simple self-massage techniques that target the trigger points of pain and common areas of tightness in and around your joints to help promote a greater sense of ease in your body and feelings of improved overall well-being. The objective in SMR is to apply mechanical stimulation to your muscles and fascia in order to facilitate deep tissue release, restore tissue pliability and resilience, improve circulation and tissue hydration, and trigger your body's own natural healing and repair processes to aid in muscle recovery. The stimulation you'll be applying is moderate pressure through intentional techniques—not just rolling around haphazardly looking for painful areas where you can keep "poking the bear." You want to work with the tissues and stick with levels of sensation that you're able to relax into and breathe through.

With these practices, you're also working to gently break up any collagen fibers that have adhered tissues together to restore the ability of the tissues to glide over each other. The pressure applied during SMR, when done conscientiously, can help restore the directional order and orientation of the collagen fibers in your fascia and stimulate the production of the slippery substance that keeps the tissues hydrated. When these tissues are hydrated and gliding well, the whole system works better.

Yoga

You might recognize many of the stretches in this book, as well as some of the muscular activation exercises, as things you've encountered in a yoga class. However, I haven't specifically labeled any sections as the "yoga" sections the way that I've done with corrective exercise and myofascial release work. The reason for this is

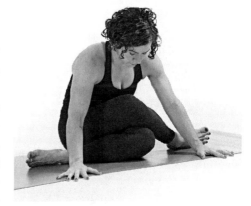

Yoga facilitates focus and self-awareness.

that I'd really like you to think of all the work in this book as yoga because all of it will give you the benefits of yoga if you are doing it mindfully.

Most people think of yoga as the poses you see in pictures, but the reality is that yoga poses are only a very small part of what yoga involves. Yoga is a philosophical approach to life that offers tools you can practice in your daily life to help you become a happier and more functional human being. *The Yoga Sutras of Patanjali* is the text that lays out the eight limbs (or practices) of yoga, which essentially provide strategies for living a more ethical, meaningful, and fulfilled life. The poses (or asana) are only one of those eight limbs and they are designed to be tools to help you be more aware of the ways you approach yourself and your life.

But here's the thing—you can do yoga poses without practicing yoga. And you can practice yoga without doing yoga poses. Your ability to perform yoga poses does not in any way interfere with or enhance your ability to benefit from the practice of yoga. There is so much more depth to the practice than how flexible you are or whether you can stand on your head. Rather than focusing on yoga as a strictly flexibility or strength modality, my goal is to get you to see yoga, and the mindfulness it brings, as a tool to create better balance in your body and improve the quality of your movement so that it's more sustainable in the long term.

You can practice yoga in everything you do. Yoga, very simply put, is what happens when you stop the fluctuations of your mind. It's what happens when you learn to separate yourself from and not be controlled by your own mental noise—your fears, your beliefs, your patterns, your feelings, your tendencies, and your doubts. It's not a specific posture or a series of poses. It's a skill, one that you can bring to any shape or activity. One that you can practice in every moment of every day. One that changes and grows and adapts with you to support you in every aspect of your life, not just the things you do within the four corners of a yoga mat.

What makes the everyday things you do a yoga practice is the awareness and intention you bring to them. You can practice while you run, while you do the dishes, while you hang out with your kids. Any time you try to create space in your head by simply focusing on the moment that you're in, you are practicing yoga. We all practice yoga from time to time—some people just don't call it that. They might call it mindfulness, self-awareness, or "flow state." But at its core, whatever you call it, it's yoga.

So when I say that yoga is an integral part of the durability training model outlined in this book, I'm not referring to specific poses. I mean that I want you to pay attention. I want you to get to know yourself better, dedicate the proper attention to recognizing your patterns (both physical and mental), and work to change them in a way that serves you better, so you can be your best self—both on the race course and off. When you're performing the work described in this book, don't just go through the motions so you can check off the boxes saying you did what you needed to do today. Pay attention to how things feel. Use the mobility time to drop into relaxation mode—get curious and notice the subtleties of what you're experiencing in your body. Use the myofascial release time to work on conditioning your nervous system to respond more appropriately to mild discomfort. Use the activation and strength work to really focus on creating more support for yourself and the way you move.

Yoga can happen anywhere. Learn to practice it out there on the pavement, at your job, and in your relationship the same way you do on your mat. If you do that, the practice suddenly becomes a lot more influential and powerful. The biggest shift for me came when I stopped only practicing yoga on my mat and instead let every moment be a chance to practice these important skills. Expect to see them woven throughout every aspect of this book.

KEY POINT: *The Eight Limbs of Yoga*

There are many ways to apply the practices of yoga to your life—and to your running. Yoga doesn't give you a prescription for how to live your best life, it simply offers the tools—how you apply them is totally up to

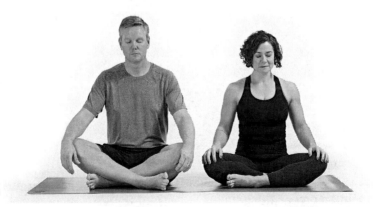

The poses are a small part of what makes up the practice of yoga.

you. When bad things happen to you in life, there's a moment between that event and your reaction to it. In that moment, you can intentionally choose to apply the practices of yoga. You have the opportunity to draw from the eight limbs to take the cards you've been dealt and turn them into something of value that moves you forward in a positive direction. Here's a brief look at the eight limbs.

1. The *Yamas* are five behaviors you should practice not doing. They are *ahimsa* (don't cause harm), *satya* (don't be dishonest), *asteya* (don't take more than is rightfully yours), *brahmacarya* (don't cross boundaries or go to extremes), and *aparigraha* (don't cling to things).

2. The *Niyamas* are five behaviors you should practice more of in your life. They are *sauca* (order and clarity), *santosa* (contentment), *tapas* (discipline), *svadhyaya* (self-study), and *isvara-pranidhana* (surrender to something or some purpose that's bigger than yourself).

3. *Asana* means "seat" and traditionally it's a term used to describe the poses you do during a yoga class. These poses are meant to help you work through any tightness and weakness in your body that might otherwise make you squirm around and prevent you from being able to sit comfortably in meditation. The idea is that if you properly care for your body and move it regularly, it will be less of distraction for you.

4. *Pranayama* is often translated as "freeing up the breath" and refers to breath work designed to help you be more aware of your breath and how much daily stress and poor postural habits have negatively affected your breathing patterns. This awareness helps you learn to breathe more efficiently and in a way that supports you and the things you do.

5. *Pratyahara* is the practice of "turning inward" and being more aware of what's going on with you instead of what's happening all around you. You're bombarded by external stimulation all day so it's good to turn the volume down on all that noise every now and then to focus on you and your needs.

6. *Dharana* is the practice of concentration—focusing your attention on one thing. In our fast-paced world, it can be a challenge to develop this skill but, when practiced consistently, this simple

practice helps you learn that you have the ability to choose where you direct your attention. That's a really powerful thing.

7. *Dhyana* is the sense of presence that comes in practices like meditation, which we'll dive deeper into later in this book. It's the ability to watch what you're feeling, thinking, and experiencing without getting tangled up in or distracted by it. It's easy to get overwhelmed by everything and this is my secret for maintaining sanity—taking a few moments to separate myself from everything long enough to find clarity and calm amidst the chaos.

8. *Samadhi* is a state where you feel a deep and meaningful connection with the world around you. When you accept that not everything is about you, the pressure of life lessens and you realize that you're not alone on this journey called life.

Embracing the Process

As with everything else in life, there are no quick fixes, no short-cuts, and no ways around consistently engaging in the process. There is no magic in the work prescribed in this book. Of course it's based on relevant, solid, and sound information as well as my experience and the experience of the athletes I've trained, but the true remedy is in the process, my friends. The work prescribed in this book will only help you if you commit to the process of recognizing your habits and patterns and take the necessary steps to change them.

Expect that some things will come faster than others. Muscles are generally the quickest to respond. Fascia is generally slower to respond, although you may feel a difference right away when we get into the SMR techniques described later in this book. But it will take time for your nervous system to wire a new movement pattern and even longer for you to cut through the mental constructs, thought patterns, and self-limiting beliefs that have accumulated throughout your life.

Durability is a lifelong process. If you picked up this book in the hopes that a couple of weeks of work following my instructions will have you free to return to business as usual, this is the part where I break the bad news. You will be in constant pursuit of balance for the rest of your life. There will always be monkey wrenches. There will always be distractions. There will always be setbacks. You have to carry on anyway.

But if you truly commit to the process, the rewards for doing so extend far beyond just your running. The qualities and characteristics gained through the process of self-study and training for durability will stay with you and will help you deal with life and all the changes it brings with grace.

How to Use This Book

There's a lot of information in this book. Don't get overwhelmed. You don't need to do every single thing in this book to reap the benefits of training for durability. A little bit of the right things, when done consistently, can go a long way. This book will give you lots of new tools for your toolbox and walk you through different ways that you can use these tools to develop an effective solution for yourself that fits into your life.

For the sake of simplicity, I have made some generalizations in this book, but each of us is very different. Some people are really strong in some places and weaker in others. The key is to use this information as a guide to help you figure out where to focus your efforts for maximum impact. Durability training begins with recognizing your own natural tendencies and consciously developing the things that aren't as easy for you.

As you work your way through the next parts, rather than looking at all the prescribed mobility, self-myofascial release (SMR), and corrective exercises as boxes you need to check every day, explore them to find which have the biggest impact for you. You can and should skip the things you're already good at and spend more time on the things that are most difficult, foreign, or uncomfortable for you—because the movements and positions you struggle with are the biggest opportunities for improvement. Injuries are often an indication of some sort of imbalance. Therefore, in order to break the cycle of injury, you're looking for ways to move yourself closer to balance. You don't have to do it all, you just have to find and do the things that move the dial for you the most. This book will be your guide in that process.

What to Expect

The exercise portion of this book is broken down into parts by section of the body so you can easily zero in on and troubleshoot your specific area of concern. The sooner you're able to identify the things that are the real game-changers for you, the quicker you can put them into action and the faster you'll start to feel better. And that is my goal—to make it easier for you to feel better sooner.

Each part begins with a brief introduction to the subject region. We'll explore why it's important, what the demands of running require, and what the typical major challenges are. We'll also look at some of the ways that injury can develop in that area before we dive into the relevant anatomy and physiology.

Knowledge is power. When you understand your anatomy, it doesn't feel so mysterious and overwhelming anymore. Your body starts to feel more familiar to you. You learn how to respond to it with compassion. Additionally, the more you know about your body, the more you realize that everything in it is happening for a reason. And the real "trick" (if there is one here) is to address the underlying reason that things are happening rather than just continuing to insist on running through them—especially because more mileage is not usually the answer.

The more you know about what's happening in your body, the more options you'll have to move forward. Understanding the anatomical structures and their functions is the key to skillfully and effectively troubleshooting when things don't feel quite right. You wouldn't take your laptop for repairs to someone who's never studied or seen the inside of a computer before. You have to have some familiarity with the equipment and its optimal function before you can start teasing out how to address dysfunction. The anatomy and physiology parts of this book are designed to give you options: options to improve your resiliency to prevent injury, options to improve your running form to become more powerful, options to fine-tune the way you move to be more effective, and options to better posture or position yourself to stop the reoccurrence of those nagging aches and pains.

After we've looked at the anatomical structures and how they should be functioning together to support you as you run, we'll spend some time talking about the most common issues among runners. Then we'll lay out the objectives for the work that follows, so it's clear what we're trying to accomplish and why it's so important. This is where you'll get specific directives that will form your roadmap to creating more durability for yourself.

While this book is designed for navigational simplicity and ease, I also highly recommend you consider the parts referencing regions both above and below your specific area of concern. Everything in your body is connected. Some issues are caused by something upstream or downstream from where the pain and discomfort shows up. For example, pain in your knee could be the result of instability in your foot or limited ankle range of motion (the joints below your knees) or areas of tightness or weakness in your hips (the joint above your knees). While you will naturally zero in on your specific areas of concern, be sure to broaden your view for best results.

The Movement Practices

In each part of this book, there are three movement practices designed to help you restore balance—one for mobility, one for SMR, and one outlining corrective activation and strengthening work. Your first few times through the work prescribed in each part should be more exploratory. Do all the work listed and notice what feels great and what feels more challenging as well as what comes easily to you and what does not.

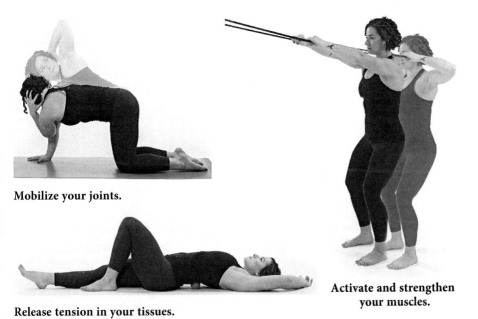

Mobilize your joints.

Release tension in your tissues.

Activate and strengthen your muscles.

After a few times through it, you'll recognize the things that would be the most valuable for you to repeat regularly and have a pretty good idea of where to focus your efforts. Most of us don't need more things added to our to-do lists. Aim to be as efficient as possible with your time and establish a practice that moves you closer to balance, not further away.

Once you've identified the work that offers the most potential for improvement for you, you'll create customized regular movement practices that meet your specific needs, taking into consideration how much time you have available. The practices do not have to be done at the same time, in a certain order, or in their entirety. Slice and dice it up in any way that makes sense. Feel free to combine the work into one session or sprinkle pieces of it throughout your day or your week. Play with the order and time of day that you do them and see what offers you the most benefit. I've had great success stringing some of the movements together to make short but effective pre-run warm-ups and post-run cool downs for my athletes. I personally also love to use five or six of the movements every day as part of a short morning routine for myself and then just alternate the work every other day or so based on what I'm feeling. But there really are no rules. Find something that works well for you and fits into your life so it's sustainable in the long term. I'll provide more ideas for how to make durability training work for you in the final chapters of this book.

These movement practices are designed to help you connect to the communities of muscles through sensation and awareness. While it may be tempting only to consult this book and do the prescribed work at times when you're feeling the effects of imbalance, you'll likely find the real benefit of it is to prevent imbalance from reoccurring—which means that you need to stay ahead of it. A little bit of something every day is optimal—even if it's just 10 minutes to start or end your day.

The Mobility Practices

The mobility work in this book should put you in a position where your tissues can relax and release. You should not be white-knuckling your way through this stuff, and it shouldn't be a lot of effort for you to hold the positions. With this work, you're looking for something that feels like a mild to moderate stretch—a sensation your body can gradually soften around.

Think of it this way: if someone obsessively and aggressively pulled on your arm all the time, would you relax? Probably not. The tissues in your body probably won't release under those circumstances either. If aggressive stretching was a good long-term solution for what's happening in your body, it would have worked already, don't you think? Instead, let's try a softer approach for these chronically tight areas that might allow them to chill out a bit. Learn to do less.

The Self-Myofascial Release Practices

Similar to the mobility work above, in terms of sensation, you're looking for intensities that are manageable when doing SMR. Expect this work to be uncomfortable, but it should not be painful. You should still be able to breathe in a relaxed way. SMR is not punishment for your tissues, and you shouldn't be treating it that way. Gentler is often better.

Don't be afraid to explore the tissues in these areas a little—move around slowly and carefully, applying light to moderate pressure at first, and let sensation be your guide. Avoid anything that feels painful, sharp, shooting, or radiates outward. If you do encounter a painful spot, rather than staying there and trying to drive the myofascial balls in deeper, move just slightly off the spot to the nearby tissues. If you're working with tissues that are already a bit sore, I recommend going indirect before direct—start with the nearby tissues before heading for the site of your pain. For areas that are especially tender, it might make more sense for you to stand up and do the techniques at a wall where you can moderate the pressure more easily.

You don't have to spend a lot of time doing SMR. In fact, I favor frequency over duration. A little bit done more often is generally far more effective than long sessions that are rarely done. I plan for 10 minutes of SMR every evening—it's a great way to unwind before bed.

You should not be significantly sore after SMR. I know people who have gotten overzealous and given themselves bruises—that's not what you're looking for. If you find that you're pretty sore after doing SMR, ease up a bit next time. SMR triggers inflammation, which can be helpful for healing, but you don't want to go digging around in vulnerable tissues and irritate them.

One final pro tip on the SMR presented in this book: in between each technique, take a few moments to lie still on your back to notice the effects of the SMR work. You might notice a change in temperature or sensation to the tissues you just worked with or a subtle feeling of rein-vigoration there as the circulation returns. You might even notice that the surrounding tissues feel different. Sometimes what you feel is even more subtle than that. You might notice the subtleties the most on single-sided work if you pause to lie on your back for a moment between sides. You might feel that one side feels bigger than the other side or that one side feels closer to the ground. You might not even be able to put your finger on what feels different, but do take a few moments to pause and notice how you feel after—if for no other reason than to notice if there is some effect for you. Why continue to spend time on practices that don't make a difference for you?

The Corrective Strengthening Practices

Ultimately, you want a community of muscles that is active and able to do its job to provide 360 degrees of support around your joints. With the corrective strength work in this book, you'll learn simple, targeted exercises to help activate and build strength in your stabilizer muscles for proper joint support. The focus will be primarily on these smaller and deeper muscles, and for that reason, corrective exercise is not designed to take the place of higher-resistance strength training, where the focus is on your bigger, more superficial mover muscles. In fact, when done consis-tently, the corrective work in this book should help amplify the effects of your regular resistance training, since stability is a precursor for powerful and efficient movement.

Equipment

All of the stretches, techniques, and exercises presented in this book are simple things you can do at home with minimal space and equipment to supplement your other training. This is by design. I know that if I can do the work at home in my lounging clothes, it's more likely to actually happen. Not having to drive to the gym or needing a shower after getting sweaty makes durability training a bit easier to accomplish on a regular basis, which makes it more likely to become habit.

Each movement practice within each part specifies what is needed for that specific practice so you can have the equipment and props nearby before you get started. But generally, here's what you want to have on hand to get the most out of this book:

- Two yoga blocks (either foam or cork blocks will work fine)
- A yoga strap (or a belt)
- A blanket (or some bath towels)
- A bolster (or a stack of pillows, blankets, or towels will work)
- A rolled-up yoga mat (a rolled-up blanket could substitute as well)
- A kitchen towel or a carpet slider disc

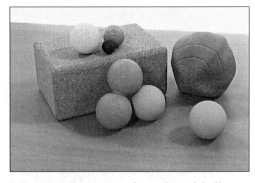

Have an assortment of myofascial balls handy.

- A foam roller (a rolled-up blanket could substitute as well)
- A few myofascial release balls of different sizes—such as the RAD Rounds and RAD Recovery Rounds (lacrosse or tennis balls can be substituted for most of the SMR work, but having a few smaller balls of different sizes will be helpful)
- A double myofascial release ball—such as the RAD Roller (or put two myofascial balls in a long sock and tie off the end)
- Some mini resistance bands (Thera-Bands tied into a small loop would also work)
- A long thin resistance band (Thera-Bands tied into a big loop work for this)
- A piece of PVC pipe or a dowel that is at least as wide as your shoulders

Running Form Notes

Each part wraps up with notes on running form. These cues transfer to your running the knowledge and self-awareness that you'll gain by reading through and implementing the prescribed work. The goal is to help you run better, so we need to apply this knowledge and awareness during your runs. Consistent mobility, SMR, and corrective work on the areas where you're struggling will help you connect with your running muscles in a new way. There's no better time to experience what it's like to support yourself well than by going for a run to feel it out.

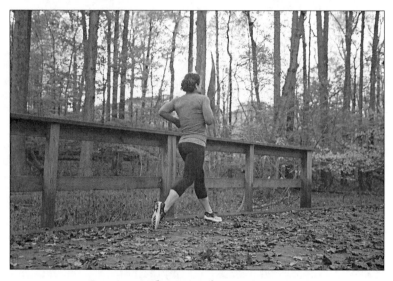

Practice good running form on every run.

I also encourage you to think of each run as form practice. The things you practice are the things you continue doing. If you let your form fade during hard efforts or during the final miles of your longer runs, you're reinforcing patterns that ultimately could continue feeding the cycle of injury and dysfunction and wreck your chances of improving your running times.

Making It Work for You

As a runner, you're probably already accustomed to following a specific weekly routine or training schedule. I encourage you to do the same with the material in this book. It's not always easy to find the time to squeeze supplemental injury-prevention work into an already-packed life.

The final chapters of this book will help you break it down and make it manageable for you. Know that you don't have to do it all every day or even every other day for it to help. Rather than thinking of it as a complete system overhaul that you have to tackle all at once, think of it as just a bunch of little things you do every day to move the dial just a little bit more.

Take the time to identify the things that have the potential to create the biggest impact for you so that you're realistically able to do the work with regularity. Think shorter and more frequent practices rather than long marathon sessions that you're only able to squeeze into your life once in a blue moon. Brief practices done consistently can add up to significant gains. We're not in a rush here. Working with your body to make positive changes will take time. Be patient with yourself.

Working through Injury

This is a book about developing resiliency and preventing injury. My assumption is that many people will pick it up because they are injured and cannot train either at the level they would like or at all. So let's talk about working through injury.

First and foremost, when in doubt, speak to your healthcare provider. Nothing in this book should be considered a substitute for sound advice from a medical professional who is aware of your unique injury concerns and history. Seek medical guidance and then follow it. Be smart, people.

Here is the general guidance that I give my athletes and students when they show up injured. It's a two-part inquiry. First, I ask my athlete or student what he or she is experiencing: (a) a dull, achy, and generalized pain, (b) pain on both sides of your body, or (c) pain in the belly of the muscle (meaning not close to a joint)? Or is it (a) a sharp pain that is (b) in a very specific location (meaning you could point to the exact spot with one or two fingers) which is (c) on or near a joint and (d) only on one side of your body? If it's the former, then you're probably okay to move on to part two of this inquiry. If it's the latter, I would say steer clear of work that directly affects that joint and stick only to movements that you can do pain-free. Second, I have a 10-minute rule: if after 10 minutes of gentle movement, the discomfort lessens and you feel better, give the workout a go and be mindful of how you feel throughout. However, if during that first 10 minutes of gentle movement the discomfort worsens or does not improve at all, it's time to stop.

Regardless of how you proceed, when you're dealing with an injury, it's usually better to work indirectly before directly. If your lower back is achy, start by working your hips and shoulders (the areas above and below) first and see how you feel before you start in with spine and core work. The goal is greater self-awareness and developing the ability to receive feedback from your body in order to make better decisions about its well-being. Move slowly and deliberately. Notice how you feel and be compassionate to yourself.

Part 1: Feet and Lower Legs

If I were to ask you which part of a runner's body is the most important to strengthen and mobilize well, odds are you wouldn't immediately say feet and lower legs. While all runners are different and vary greatly in terms of areas of concern, I have yet to meet a runner who wouldn't benefit greatly from spending more time down here.

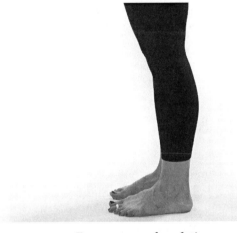

Focus on your foundation.

Your feet, ankles, and lower legs are your foundation, yet often this base is overlooked. Most runners don't include foot and ankle work in their training, but the stability and mobility in these areas set the stage for everything above. Imbalance here can have a global impact and cause all sorts of issues from your toes to your spine. While you might look at the parts of your body that are hurting the most and blame them, the underlying problem can often be traced back to a lack of stability in your feet and a lack of mobility in your ankles. Over the years, multiple runners have come to me after a full round of physical therapy with unresolved long-term hip and lower back pain and, in many of these athletes, foot-stabilization training and greater awareness of their foot strike and arch support was enough to get them running pain-free again.

There is no way around using your feet and ankles in running. They are the first places to make contact with the ground and therefore your first line of defense to absorb impact and distribute force throughout your body. They also play a key role in how powerfully and efficiently you're able to push off the ground. The major joints in your feet and ankles work together both to stabilize and to propel your running stride, and they set the tone for the alignment of your entire skeleton. You must make them durable to run well.

If the muscles in your feet are weak, they support you less, which increases the demand on your ankles, knees, and hips. Your feet must plant on the ground properly, absorb the impact of your foot strike, and quickly bounce back and push off powerfully to propel you forward with every step. The ability of the soft tissues in your feet and ankles to store and then release energy—similar to a spring—helps you to run efficiently. If your feet and ankles are not properly cared for, you lose the benefit of this ability as more of the work gets transferred to other joints upstream. This can ultimately lead to the development of aches and pains in your knees, hips, and/or lower back.

Stable feet and mobile ankles are important for everyone, but their importance for runners cannot be overstated. Running is a single-leg activity: with every foot strike, only one of your feet is contacting the ground at a time. Therefore, each of your feet and ankles independently needs to be able to absorb the weight of your entire body with every step.

Above your ankles, the muscles in your calves and shins are important for a powerful and effective running gait as well as shock absorption. Imbalance here can create problems in the joints above—the knees—and below—the ankles. Improper force application from overly-tight or constricted muscles in this area can have far-reaching consequences in your body.

If you just cram your feet into shoes all day and forget about them and your ankles, you are training the bigger, fancier stuff but forgetting to train the foundation. You need your feet and ankles to be able to adjust and conform to uneven terrain to keep you balanced and upright while supporting your body weight as well as absorb impact and transfer ground reaction forces. It's a lot to ask of body parts that you don't train regularly.

Anatomy and Physiology Basics

The Foot

You have 26 bones in each of your feet. When you add the bones of both feet together, this accounts for almost a quarter of all the bones in your body. These bones support the entire weight of your body and play a major role in your ability to walk and run. The numerous joints in your feet need to be mobile enough to adjust for a variety of surfaces but also need to be stable in order to provide a solid base for the rest of your body.

Two of the most important bones in your feet when it comes to force transmission and distribution are your heel bone (calcaneus) and your talus, which sits directly on top of your heel bone. The joint where these two bones come together is called the subtalar joint. This joint gives your foot the ability to rock from side to side and allows your foot to adjust for uneven ground.

On the bottom of your foot, from your heel all the way out to each of your individual toes, is a thick band of fibrous tissue called the plantar fascia. This piece of tissue is the support structure for the big inner arch of your foot that gives your foot the ability to act like a spring. Every time you take a step, your plantar fascia is stretched a bit as your inner arch flattens to absorb the force of impact. This tough piece of tissue is designed more for support than for flexibility, so it may become strained, develop small tears, and/or become inflamed in runners due to the repetitive stretching of the tissue as it's loaded with the weight of your body with every step. This condition is called plantar fasciitis.

Foot Movements

Healthy, balanced feet are able to both invert and evert. Inversion occurs when you turn the bottom of your foot toward the midline of your body. Eversion is the opposite, turning the sole of your foot away from the midline of your body. These joint actions are functions of the subtalar joint and play an important role in pronation and supination, both critical elements of a well-balanced gait cycle.

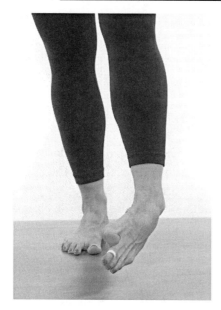 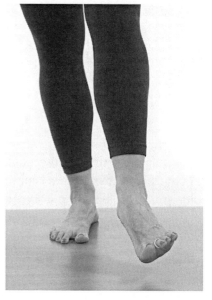

Foot Inversion.   **Foot Eversion.**

The Ankle

Your ankle joint (talocrural joint) is where your foot and lower leg come together. It's formed by three bones: your shinbone (tibia), your calf bone (fibula), and the talus in your foot. Since the ankle joint is situated directly above the subtalar joint in your foot, and both joints involve the talus, these two joints work together to give you the ability to move your foot and ankle in all directions—a capability that comes in quite handy when running or walking on uneven surfaces.

If you take a look down at your ankle, you'll notice that you have an inner ankle bone and an outer ankle bone. Your inner ankle bone is called the medial malleolus. It's really just the bottom of your shinbone, which sits on top of the talus and pokes out the side a little there. Your outer ankle bone is called the lateral malleolus. It's the bottom of your calf bone, which sits right beside your talus.

In runners, the ankle joint needs to be both mobile and stable. There are a number of ligaments that surround and support your ankles to help provide that much-needed stability. When the muscles that cross the ankle are strong, your ankle is able to withstand greater force.

ANKLE MOVEMENTS

Your ankle joint functions as a hinge joint to perform two movements:

- Plantarflexion: occurs when you point your toes
- Dorsiflexion: occurs when you pull the top of your foot back toward your shin

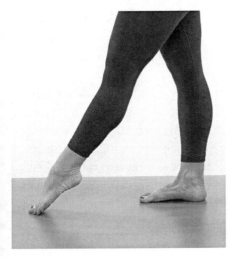 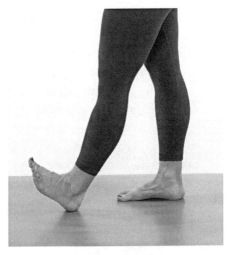

Ankle Plantarflexion.   Ankle Dorsiflexion.

KEY POINT: *Pronation and Supination*

In the running world, you often hear about pronation and supination of the feet as bad things that should be avoided. However, despite what you may have read in a magazine or heard in a running store, both pronation and supination are completely normal and necessary movements. They are specific combinations of joint actions that naturally occur as part of the gait cycle.

Pronation is a combination of eversion in your subtalar joint, dorsiflexion in your ankle, and rotation of your foot away from the midline of your body. All of these occur simultaneously as your foot makes contact with the ground and are intended to direct more of the weight of your body toward your big toe.

Supination is a combination of inversion of your subtalar joint, plantarflexion in your ankle, and rotation of your foot toward the midline of your body. All of these occur simultaneously as your foot begins the push-off phase in order to prepare for a well-balanced push off.

Both have a place in the gait cycle, and it's all about timing. Problems occur when you're doing one thing but you really should be doing the other. Sometimes this happens when you just keep on pronating instead of supinating to transfer the weight of your body to be more evenly balanced across the whole foot. Some people pronate more than is functional, which can ultimately be a little bit dysfunctional. Some people just supinate and never really roll inward for that initial pronation phase, leaving the smaller toes to absorb more impact.

There are many reasons why these things might occur—too many to unpack here. Overpronation, in particular, tends to get blamed for a lot of overuse injuries, and while there definitely seems to be some correlation, there also seems to be more to it than that since some runners overpronate without injury. In other words, there really isn't much need to worry about it unless you're experiencing injuries. If that's you, work with a podiatrist and/or physical therapist to develop a course of action to treat and prevent future issues.

The Foot and Lower Leg Muscles

You have a large number of relatively tiny bones in your feet and ankles; they give you the ability to move around in all the ways you can. Lots of small bones means lots of joints, and that means lots of ligaments, which provide some passive stability. In addition to all those ligaments, there are many muscles in your feet and ankles that all work to support you and propel you while you're running.

Let's start at the bottom with your feet. You have many muscles here—too many to name without putting you to sleep—all of which play a role in the movement of your feet and toes. Primarily, these muscles have the job of flexing and extending your toes as well as squeezing and spreading your toes and lifting the arches of your feet. Their most critical role is helping you balance. These muscles are making microadjustments any time you're standing on your feet in order to help you stabilize your whole body in space, which means that you need these little guys to be strong and able to control the movement of all the individual joints in your feet.

While the foot is built to provide stability, the ankle is designed for mobility. This becomes obvious when you take a look at the musculature that supports it. Most of the muscles that give stability to your ankles begin and end in your lower legs and feet and it's actually mostly the tendons of these muscles that cross your ankle joints and provide support. Absent appropriate mobility in your ankles, your knee (the joint right above) might be forced to move a bit more, causing an increased risk of destabilization in order to compensate, which you really don't want. But it doesn't stop there—the less stable your knee is, the stiffer your hips tend to get, which leads to lower back pain and lots of other problems upstream.

There are many muscles located in the lower leg—some you've probably heard of (like the gastrocnemius) and others maybe not so much (like the peroneals). Traditionally, these muscles are divided into categories or compartments based on function and how they are bundled by fascia encasements.

1. Anterior Compartment: These are the muscles of the front of your shin. The main job of this group is to draw your toes back and your ankle up into dorsiflexion. They also help turn your foot inward (inversion), which is how you're able to keep your shin vertical when you're running on uneven terrain.

2. Lateral Compartment: These are the muscles on the outer portion of your lower leg. This group turns your foot outward (eversion), which is the action necessary to stabilize your outer ankle when weight bearing. They also assist with pointing your toes (plantarflexion).

3. Superficial Posterior Compartment: These muscles are the ones at the back of your lower leg that give your calves their signature shape and all come together at the bottom to form the Achilles tendon (the strongest tendon in your body), which attaches to your heel bone. This is the group that helps you point your toes (plantarflexion) and, when running, powers the push-off phase of your gait cycle.

4. Deep Posterior Compartment: These muscles live deep in the back of your calves and pass behind your inner ankle bone into the bottom of your foot. They assist in plantarflexion, help curl your toes under, pull your foot inward into inversion, and provide critical support for the inner arch of your foot any time you're weight bearing on your feet.

Common Issues Among Runners

Most runners pay shockingly little attention to their feet and ankles. The few that I've met who do spend time focusing on these areas usually have a story to tell about an injury that led them to take the health of their feet and ankles more seriously. Often, that seems to be a common thread throughout the body—people don't really think about the complexity of their moving parts until there's pain involved.

Running requires a balance of strength and flexibility in the community of muscles around your feet and ankles. Your foot works hard to stabilize you with every step, and your ankle needs to move freely to keep you balanced and moving forward. These two groups work together to create a foundation that ideally allows the force absorbed and generated by running to be properly distributed throughout your body. If you lack the appropriate amount of foot stability and/or ankle mobility, the surrounding structures pay the price.

Since this area requires such a specific balance of both stability and mobility, there are a number of common running-related injuries that plague runners here. When your foot lacks stability, the plantar fascia can get strained from being repeatedly stretched while supporting the weight of your body, resulting in inflammation—a condition known as plantar fasciitis. Weakness in the muscles of your feet and lower legs may result in instability, which can set you up for ankle sprains as your ligaments have to absorb more of the work to stabilize the bones. If your ankles aren't able to move well, the force of impact gets transferred to your knees, which will ultimately make them very unhappy. Tightness in your calves can limit the mobility of your ankles but it can also irritate your Achilles tendon, which may lead to tendonitis and potentially even tendon damage.

How to Fix It

In this section, we'll focus on (1) mobilizing the tissues that cross over and support your ankles; (2) applying some compression to the tissues that have a tendency to become strained in order to stimulate circulation and reoxygenation in these areas; and (3) connecting with, activating, and strengthening the muscles of your feet and lower legs so they are better able to tolerate load and generate force.

The Movement Practices

Mobilize and Release Your Feet and Lower Legs

If you're like most runners, your poor feet probably spend a lot of time crammed into shoes and your calves have a tendency to feel a little stiff. So we're going to work on that a bit. The mobilization work that follows is designed to free up these tissues that work so hard to support you—not just in your running but also in your life.

EQUIPMENT/PROPS NEEDED: A rolled-up yoga mat or blanket.

TOE SEPARATOR WITH FOOT AND ANKLE CIRCLES

Sit in a comfortable position where you can grab your right foot and rest it on your left thigh or a block. Place the palm of your left hand on the bottom of your right foot and insert one finger between each of your toes. Give the ball of your feet and your toes a gentle squeeze. For the first round, don't move your ankle as you circle the upper part of your foot—it won't go far without moving your ankle but do what you can. Take 5 circles in one direction and then 5 circles in the other direction. For the second round on your right foot, let your ankle move freely as you circle 5 more times in one direction and then 5 times the other direction. Then switch feet and repeat.

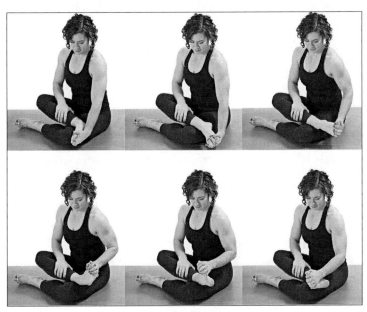

Toe Separator with Foot and Ankle Circles.

TOE SQUAT

From hands and knees, tuck your toes under and start to walk your hands back toward your knees to bring the weight of your body over your feet. As you move further into the position and begin to sit upright, this can be very intense on your toes and arches of your feet, but it should not be painful in these areas or in your knees. Take your time, ease into it, and don't force it. Feel free to keep your hands on the floor or on your knees as you lean slightly forward to decrease the intensity of the sensation in your toes and feet to something that you can stick with and relax into. If you experience knee pain in this position, try the chair option shown below and described below instead. Stay here for 5 breaths.

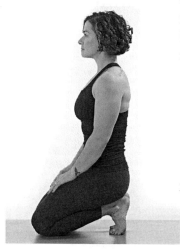

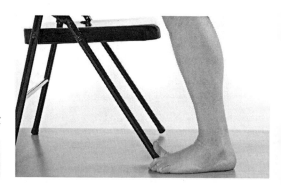

Toe Squat.   Modified Version Using a Chair.

There are several variations of this stretch that you could try in order to meet the tissues where they are and not cause pain in the joints of your legs. Here are a few options to make this one work for you:

- Work on one side at a time
- Add more support by using props—like some blocks or a bolster—under your knees which will decrease the demand on your big toe joint
- Use a chair leg or similar angled surface to get the same big toe mobilization work in without adding so much pressure to your feet, ankles, and knees

TOP OF ANKLE STRETCH

From hands and knees, place your right foot on the floor directly beside your left knee. Untuck your left toes so that the top of your left foot is on the floor and sit back so that your left hip is over your left heel. Don't let your left foot roll inward—keep your left foot pointing straight back from your ankle. If this feels like a

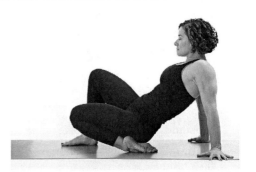

Top of Ankle Stretch.

stretch to the front of your shin and ankle already, stay there. If the stretch is mild, place your hands on the floor behind you, lean into them, and try to lift your left knee away from the floor without sickling at your left ankle. If this position bothers your left knee, come out of it and sit on the floor and use your hands to create the stretch by curling your toes under and pulling them back toward your heel. Hold for 5–10 breaths and switch sides.

CALF SMASH

Roll up a yoga mat or a blanket so that it's a couple of inches thick and make sure it's rolled tightly so it feels firm and doesn't compress

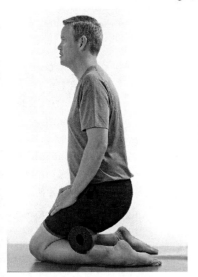

Calf Smash.

much. Come to a kneeling position with your toes untucked so that the tops of your feet are on the floor. Place the mat or blanket over the backs of your calves as close as possible to the backs of your knees. Separate your feet a bit so that your knees are closer together than your heels and sit back. It should feel a bit like you're smashing your calf muscles into your shinbones. Stay for 30 seconds and keep your breathing as relaxed as possible. Then, move the mat or blanket down about an inch or two toward your heels so that you're in the middle of your calves and repeat. Finally, move the mat or blanket another inch or two lower so you're on the bottom edge of the meaty part of your calves. Avoid this if it bothers your knees and instead do the self-myofascial release work prescribed later in this section for your calves.

TABLE/DOWN DOG CALF STRETCH

Come to your hands and knees with your wrists under your shoulders and your knees under your hips. Extend your left leg behind you with the ball of your left foot on the floor. Press into your hands and lean your weight back as you stretch your left heel back. Try this stretch both with your left leg straight and with a bent knee—spend 30 seconds or so in the variation that feels tighter. Reset and repeat on your right side. For a deeper stretch, try this stretch from a Downward-Facing Dog position: from all fours, lift your knees and press your hips up and back. Bend your right knee deeply and press your left heel toward the floor. Then switch sides.

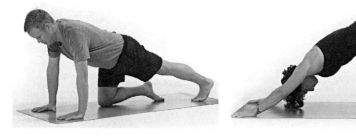

Table Calf Stretch.   Down Dog Calf Stretch.

Roll and Release Your Feet and Lower Legs

The goal here is to bring some much-needed circulation back to these tissues. We'll accomplish this by applying some mechanical stimulation in the form of moderate compression and light rolling. Know that applying pressure to the bottom of your feet can be uncomfortable—especially if this is new to you—but it should not be painful. You're looking to find a manageable amount of pressure and sensation so you get the blood flowing in to reoxygenate and reinvigorate the tissues here without sending shock waves through your whole body.

EQUIPMENT/PROPS NEEDED: a few myofascial release balls (different sizes if you have them), a double ball (optional), and a yoga block.

FEET

Stand with a medium or small myofascial release ball a few inches in front of your left foot. Keep your right foot where it is and place the center of your left foot on the ball. With most of your weight still in your right foot, shift a little bit more of your weight into your left foot and then ease up again. Repeat that a few times, leaning in and out while keeping the ball in the center—from front to back and side to side—of your left foot. This will likely be uncomfortable but it should not be painful. Then, after a few rounds of leaning in and out, pause with medium pressure on the ball and breathe. Move the ball a little to the right of where it was so that it's in the center of your outer arch on the pinky toe side of your left foot. Lean in and out again a few times then pause at medium pressure and breathe. Repeat

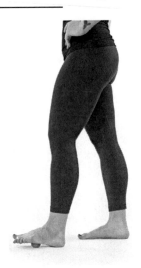

Feet SMR https:// youtu.be/LZcYPC5 Eg5U

these steps with the ball in the center of your inner arch on the big toe side of your left foot. Then, finish up on your left foot by rolling at light to medium pressure in one direction from the ball of your foot to your heel. Repeat on your right foot.

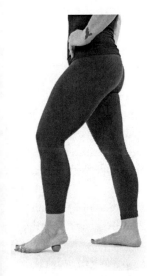

Heels SMR https://you tu.be/LZcYPC5Eg5U

HEELS

First, we'll work on the soft tissue attachment at the front of your heel bone. Stand with a medium or small myofascial release ball a few inches in front of your left foot. Keep your right foot where it is and place your left heel on top of the ball. Roll your left foot slightly back over the ball so that the ball ends up right at the front edge of your heel bone—near where your arch connects to your heel bone. Rest the ball of your left foot on the floor and try to relax your toes as much as possible. Lean a little of your weight into your left foot and rock your right heel from side to side over that connection site where your arch and heel bone come together. It might feel gritty or fibrous. Spend about 30 seconds there rocking your left heel from side to side with a tolerable amount of pressure on the ball.

Next, move the ball back so that your left heel sits directly on top of the ball, with the ball of your left foot resting on the floor and toes relaxed. Lean a little of your weight into your left foot and move your heel around over the ball. Spend about 15 seconds on your left heel and then switch feet and repeat both steps on your right foot.

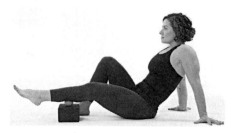

Calves SMR https://youtu.be/2lTiZ vdlM90

Calves

Sit on the floor and place a myofascial ball on top of a yoga block right in front of you. Rest your left calf on top of the ball. Place your hands on the floor behind you and lean back. Keep your left leg heavy on the ball and move your left calf around a little over the surface of the ball. For more pressure, you can cross your right leg over the top of your left leg. Once you find a spot that feels tender, pause there for a few breaths. You can also pause in any tender spot you find while circling your left ankle or pointing and flexing your left foot. Spend about a minute or two on your left leg, working up toward your left knee and down in the direction of your left heel. Switch sides and repeat.

Outer Calves

Sit on the floor with your right leg extended and your left knee bent with your left foot flat on the floor. Drop your left knee over to the left

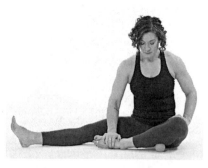

side so that the outside of your left leg is resting on the floor. Tuck a myofascial release ball under the outer edge of your upper left calf. Move your left calf around a little over the surface of the ball and once you find a spot that feels tender, pause there for a few breaths. Spend about a minute or two on your left leg, working up toward your left knee and down in the direction of your left heel. Switch sides and repeat.

Outer Calves https://youtu.be/ 0qjqr7PNfVg

SHINS

Come to your hands and knees with your wrists under your shoulders and your knees under your hips. Sit your hips back onto your heels. Place a double myofascial ball or pair of myofascial balls side by side, one on either side of your shinbone, under your left shin near your left knee. Place your hands on the floor (or yoga blocks) for support. Lean your left shin into the balls and slowly start to work your way down your left shin, pausing for a few breaths in any places that feel especially tender. Spend about a minute or two on your left leg. Switch sides and repeat.

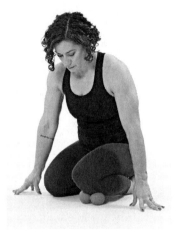

Shin MFR https://youtu.be/ yq6osjvJiUY

Balance and Strengthen Your Feet and Lower Legs

In this section, we'll work on activating and strengthening the muscles in your feet and lower legs that stabilize your arches and ankles. We'll begin by waking the small muscles in your feet up so that they are able to provide the stable foundation your body needs in order to support your running. If you can get these guys online and working for you, it'll take the pressure off your plantar fascia and all your other joints.

Then, we'll layer in some work that helps to strengthen the muscles in your lower legs that help maintain the shape of your arches and support your ankles. These tissues are critical for creating stability, fluidity, and power during the foot-strike and push-off phases of your gait cycle.

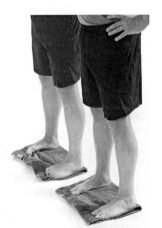

EQUIPMENT/PROPS NEEDED: a kitchen towel, a mini band, a stack of pillows (or a foam pad), and a step (or a yoga block).

TOWEL SCRUNCH

Stand (or sit in a chair) with your feet on a kitchen towel. Stretch and splay your toes out and then use them to scrunch up the towel as if you were trying to pick it up with your toes.

Towel Scrunch.

Keep your ankles neutral so they don't roll outward. You might experience some cramping as you do this the first few times—if that happens just back off and shake out your toes before trying again. This one also takes some practice since these are muscles that tend to be neglected—it'll get easier with practice. Perform 3 sets of 8–10 reps.

Arch Crunches

Stand with the soles of your feet on a kitchen towel. Curl all of your toes up away from the floor and press down into the base of your big toes as you draw them back toward your heel as if to lift and shorten the arch of your foot. The fabric under your feet will crinkle up a bit in the space between the balls of your feet and your heels—this is helpful feedback since the lifting of your arch will be subtle. The goal is to get your arches to engage and lift a little without sickling or rolling outward at your ankles— your shins should remain at a right angle to your feet. Perform 3 sets of 8–10 reps. For this exercise, consider doing one

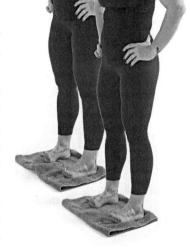

Arch Crunches https://youtu.be/ duYlz4sh-h4

foot at a time until you get the hang of it since the movement is subtle and often challenging at first. Once you master toes up variation, try it while keeping your toes down but relaxed.

Mini Band Doming

This one is similar to the Arch Crunches above but we're adding a little resistance. Place a mini band around or just above your ankles. Try to keep your toes as relaxed as possible as you lift and shorten the arches of your feet. This will create a dome-shaped space under your arches that comes from the muscles in the soles of your feet engaging and not from your ankles rolling outward. Squeeze and relax. Perform 3 sets of 8–10 reps.

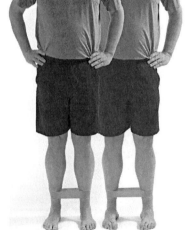

Mini Band Doming https://youtu.be/4swmp MWCY2o

Mini Band Inversion Pulls

Sit comfortably on the floor with your right leg extended in front of you (knee straight or bent is fine). Place one end of a mini band around the ball of your foot and hold the other end of the band with your right hand just to the outside of your right leg. Working against the tension of the band, using only your foot and ankle, pull the band as you turn the bottom of your foot toward the midline of your body. Perform 3 sets of 8–10 reps per foot.

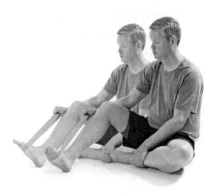

Mini Band Inversion Pulls https://youtu.be/BlVzO5O7ZnM

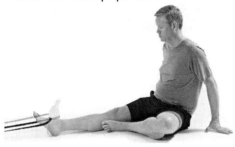

Banded Shin Pulls.

Banded Shin Pulls

Sit comfortably on the floor with your right leg extended in front of you. Anchor a long resistance band to something sturdy in front of you and place the loop just below the base of your toes over the top of your right foot. Start with a little tension on the band and working against that tension, draw the top of your foot back toward your right shin. Pause for a moment and slowly return to the start. Perform 3 sets of 8–10 reps per foot.

Heel Raises with Toe Curls

Stand with the balls of your feet on a step (heels hovering off the edge) near a wall or sturdy railing that you can hang onto for balance. Place a rolled-up towel under your toes and squeeze your toes into the towel. Take three seconds to slowly lower your heels down toward the floor as far as you're com-

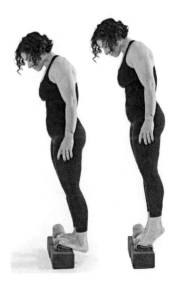

Heel Raises with Toe Curls.

fortably able. Then, take three seconds to rise up onto the balls of your feet. Pause at the top for two seconds with curled toes squeezing the towel and repeat. Perform 3 sets of 8–10 reps. Consider doing this exercise one foot at a time until you get the hang of it since the movement can be quite challenging at first.

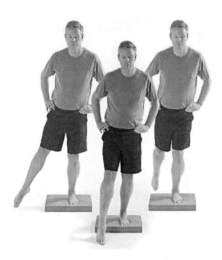

Single Leg Balancing Taps.

Single Leg Balancing Taps

Stand on an unstable surface such as a stack of pillows or a foam pad. Bend your left knee a little and keep it in line with your second and third toes. Lift your right foot and lightly tap your right toes to the floor off to your right side but don't lean or pop your left hip out to the left side. Then, tap your right toes on the floor in front of you. Finally, tap your right toes to the floor behind you and repeat. Perform 3 sets of 3 reps per foot in each direction.

Heel Walking

This one is pretty self-explanatory. Stand tall and lift your toes and the balls of your feet up away from the floor. Once you've got your balance, walk forward on your heels without lowering the balls of your feet to the floor. Perform 3 sets of 10–15 steps per foot (20–30 steps total).

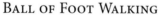

Heel Walking.

Ball of Foot Walking

Stand tall with your feet hip-width distance apart. Lift your heels and rise up onto the balls of your feet. Walk forward without letting your heels touch the floor. Perform 15 steps per leg.

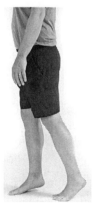

Ball of Foot Walking.

Notes on Running Form

Your feet and ankles are your first line of defense when it comes to efficiency and durability in your running stride. The things that happen here set the tone for everything that follows. Now that we've covered how to stabilize your feet and lower legs and mobilized your ankles, it's important that you take the time to pay attention to how you're contacting and pushing off the ground so you're setting yourself up for success. Let's look at some of the ways you can take these elements and transfer them to your running stride.

- **Do try to land somewhere in the middle of your foot.** Don't overthink this one. Just focus on landing somewhere between the front of your heel and your midfoot, then quickly rolling forward. The goal here is to minimize the amount of time that your foot is contacting the ground because that extended ground contact reduces the time you spend moving forward.
- **Don't strike hard and loud.** When your foot contacts the ground, it should do so relatively quietly as opposed to slapping or thudding as it strikes. Try to land softly without making a lot noise.
- **Do push off the ground like you mean it.** To run well, you need to be able to push off the ground with maximum force. As you roll forward toward your toes, try to spring off the ground and think about using and coordinating your toes and calves to powerfully propel you forward with each step.
- **Don't kick your foot out in front of you.** Focus on landing with your foot under you instead of reaching forward for the ground in front of you. If your lower leg extends out in front of your body, your stride is too long. Focus on taker shorter, but faster, steps and keep your knees slightly bent rather than kicking your lower leg forward.

Part 2: Knees and Hips

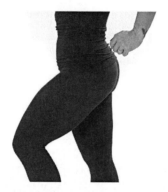

Rebalance your wheels.

The muscles of your hips and thighs are some of the largest and most powerful muscles in your body. So it's no wonder runners focus hard on these areas; after all, these are the muscles largely responsible for propelling us toward the finish line. However, the biggest challenge that runners typically face here isn't insufficient strength in the muscles that power their running stride, it's imbalance among the muscles that support and move the hip joint.

Much of your ability to run well depends on each and every muscle in the hips and thighs doing its own job and doing it well. But runners have a couple of things working against balance in and around the hips. First, no matter how many miles runners log, they still often spend many more hours every day sitting. If this is you, it's important to note that all that sitting may have conditioned your body to do the opposite of what you need it to do in order to run efficiently and without injury. Second, running is a repetitive-motion sport. With the muscles of this area of the body being the primary drivers of that repetitive movement, there is great potential here for the muscles to become unbalanced if you don't intentionally work to keep the muscles on all sides of the hip joint balanced in terms of strength and range of motion.

The hip joints are capable of moving through multiple planes of motion, but most of us typically don't train them that way. Instead, we spend large portions of the day with our hips in one position—flexed—and moving in only one plane of motion—forward and back. As a result, certain muscles around the hip begin to get tight from being in a shortened position for long periods of time, certain muscles begin to get weak from underuse, and other muscles step in to help and develop dominance. This creates imbalance, and with it the potential for dysfunction and injury.

The goal is to restore balance in the hips from front to back and side to side. This way, you can ensure that all your hip muscles are able to generate sufficient force to do their job well so others won't have to take over. You also don't want your muscles acting on the joints of the hips and knees in a way that causes the bones to be pulled out of alignment. When the bones of your joints are misaligned, they can bump into things they shouldn't, which ultimately can lead to joint damage.

Due to the repetitive nature of running in combination with postural habits, lifestyles heavy in sitting, and the unavoidable long-term effects of gravity, you see the highest concentration of muscles that are both tight and weak around the hips. This combination of tightness and weakness can lead to injury and discomfort in both the hips and the knees.

Anatomy and Physiology Basics

The Hip Joint

The hip joint is formed by two bones: your pelvis and your femur (thighbone). It's a ball and socket joint—in this case, the "ball" refers to the knob at the top of your femur and the "socket" refers to the acetabulum, a cup-shaped depression on the outer edge of your pelvis. The ball and socket nature of the hip joint makes it a joint that was designed for mobility but, when you examine the joint structures, it's clear that there's also a demand for stability here.

The acetabulum itself is deep, but the labrum (a piece of fibrocartilage attached to the acetabulum) forms a lip around the edge that extends the depth of the socket even further and creates more encapsulation to help the bones fit together snugly.

The surface of the bones that form the joint are covered by a layer of cartilage that acts as a cushion, which is lubricated with fluid produced inside the joint. This allows the femur to glide smoothly over the surface of the acetabulum so that you're not grinding bone on bone every time you take a step. The ligaments that wrap around the hip joint and form the joint capsule are some of the strongest ligaments in your body. On top of all those layers of stability are the large muscles and tendons that add another layer of joint stabilization.

HIP MOVEMENTS AND PELVIC TILT

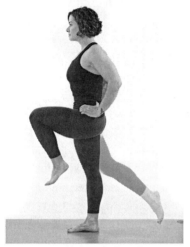

Hip Flexion and Extension.

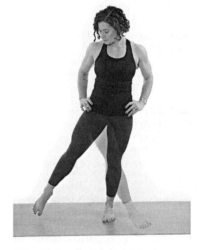

Hip Abduction and Adduction.

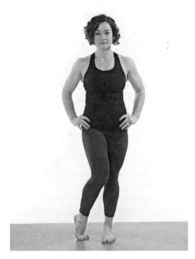

Hip Internal Rotation.

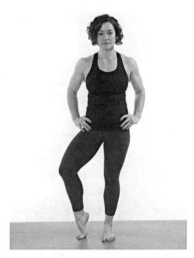

Hip External Rotation.

Healthy hips can move in six ways:

- Hip Flexion: occurs when your thigh and torso move closer together
- Hip Extension: occurs when your thigh moves back behind your torso
- Hip Abduction: occurs when your thigh moves out to the side and away from the midline of your body
- Hip Adduction: occurs when your thigh moves in toward the midline of your body
- Internal Hip Rotation: occurs when your thigh rotates inward in the socket toward the midline of your body
- External Hip Rotation: occurs when your thigh rotates outward in the socket away from the midline of your body

The above movements refer to the way that the head of your femur moves inside your acetabulum. But your whole pelvis can also move a little, which is called a tilt. This movement is defined by the position and angle of the bony points at the front of your pelvis (called the anterior superior iliac spine or "ASIS") relative to the bones at the back of your pelvis. If you were to think about your pelvis like a bowl full of marbles, angling the two ASIS points downward would spill marbles out the front of the bowl and, conversely, angling the two ASIS points upward would

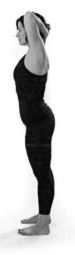 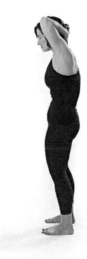

Anterior Pelvic Tilt.   **Posterior Pelvic Tilt.**

spill marbles out the back of the bowl. Somewhere in the middle of those two end-range positions is neutral.

Each of these movements are valuable, and each has implications for posture and running form. They are:

- Anterior Pelvic Tilt: occurs when you angle the ASIS points down and the back of your pelvis moves upward
- Posterior Pelvic Tilt: occurs when you angle the ASIS points up and the back of your pelvis move downward

KEY POINT: *Does Anterior Pelvic Tilt Cause Lower Back Pain?*

You may have heard that anterior pelvic tilt can lead to lower back pain, along with claims that it's caused by weak and tight muscles around the pelvis. Or you may have heard the opposite: that anterior pelvic tilt is completely normal and has no link to lower back pain.

There are three questions to ask:

1. Is anterior pelvic tilt normal?
2. What causes anterior pelvic tilt?
3. Does anterior pelvic tilt cause lower back pain?

Let's answer each.

1. Is anterior pelvic tilt normal? Yes. When looking at static posture, a 2011 study* showed that 85 percent of males and 75 percent of females have some degree of anterior pelvic tilt. Compare those numbers to their findings that 6 percent of males and 7 percent of females have posterior tilt and 9 percent of males and 18 percent of females are neutral. Clearly, exhibiting some anterior tilt to your pelvis does not make you abnormal.

2. What causes anterior pelvic tilt? We don't really know. There isn't any good scientific evidence to support the claim that it's caused by muscle tightness or weakness. It could very well be due to the shape and orientation of your bones, which varies greatly from person to person. It's possible it's a little of both and what we

*Herrington, L. (2011). *Assessment of the degree of pelvic tilt within a normal asymptomatic population.* Man Ther, 16: 646–648.

have here is a chicken vs. egg scenario—perhaps it's due to anatomical variation and some muscles are tighter or weaker as a result. Maybe it's just a postural adaptation. For now, the root cause is still unclear.

3. <u>Does anterior pelvic tilt cause lower back pain?</u> Not necessarily. First, we have to make the distinction between what is present during static posture (when you're just standing there) and what happens when you move. Studies have shown no definitive relationship between lower back pain and anterior pelvic tilt in static posture and everyday living. However, it can lead to lower back pain during running and resistance training if the degree of tilt is excessive or otherwise close to the maximum amount that your pelvis is capable of tilting anteriorly—this is referred to as your end range. In general, extreme ranges of motion for the spine and pelvis are potentially injurious when combined with impact or when under load. In other words, what might be completely safe and normal when simply standing upright might not be so helpful or appropriate when going for a run or lifting weights. And that's the case here. Runners should work to minimize excessive pelvic tilt while running, especially if they are experiencing lower back pain.

Bottom line: In static posture, some people have anterior pelvic tilt, some people have posterior pelvic tilt, and others' hips are more neutrally positioned. None of these are inherently bad or scientifically linked to lower back pain. Regardless of your natural postural inclination, we should all be able to tilt the pelvis both ways and do some degree of each. When in motion, there are certain advantages to each and there are reasons why each may create greater injury potential, but this varies based on the movement and degree of tilt. When running or lifting weights, excessive or end-range anterior pelvic tilt can lead to lower back pain or injury. Excessive pelvic tilt may be a compensation for weakness in certain muscles when performing certain movements. It's good practice to work on the tissues that affect the position of the pelvis and lumbar spine to ensure that they are not overly tense or weak. Balance is best.

The Hip Muscles

There are many powerful muscles that cross the hip joint to create movement there. In fact, part of the added stability that these large muscles provide comes from the fact that none of them connect to the joint itself. Instead, they literally cross over the joint and attach to surrounding areas close to the joint, creating a protective encasement over the joint capsule. For simplicity, let's break the hip muscles into groups based on their primary action.

First, you have the extensors. These muscles lie at the back of your hips and, as the name suggests, they draw your thighbone back and extend your hip. They are:

- Gluteus Maximus: your main hip extensor that runs from the center of the back of your pelvis to your outer thigh and IT band. It also works to draw the head of your femur slightly back in the socket so it doesn't press into the soft tissues at the front of the joint.
- Hamstrings: a group of three muscles that run from your sit bones down the back of your thigh. They assist your gluteus maximus in extending your hip.

Then, you have the hip flexors. These muscles draw your thigh and torso closer together and flex your hip. They are:

- Iliopsoas: this is actually two muscles (iliacus and psoas) with similar actions that really can't be separated. Your psoas is hooked into your lumbar spine and runs down into your hip, where it joins the iliacus—the muscle that lines the inside of the large bones of your hip (ilium)—and both muscles attach to your inner upper thighbone.
- Rectus Femoris: one of your quadriceps muscles, the only one that crosses the hip joint. This one attaches to your ASIS at the front of your pelvis and runs down the front of your thigh.

Next, you have the hip adductors. This is a group of several muscles that all work together to draw your thigh toward the midline of your body. For simplicity, we'll refer to them collectively as a group.

Let's look at the abductors. These muscles take your thigh away from the midline of your body and out to the side. They are:

- Gluteus Medius: your primary hip abductor, but it's also largely responsible for stabilizing your hip and keeping your pelvis level when you walk or run.
- Tensor Facsia Latae (TFL): does a little bit of a lot of things in

addition to assisting your gluteus medius in abduction. This muscle also connects into the top of your IT band with gluteus maximus.

Finally, there are the external rotators, which live pretty deep in the back of your pelvis under your glute muscles. These muscles also play an important role in helping to stabilize the hips and sacroiliac joint. They are:

- Piriformis: the more familiar external rotator mostly due to its proximity to the sciatic nerve.
- Deep Hip Rotators: a group of small hip rotators just below the piriformis.

While each group listed above has a specific function from which it derives its group name, they don't just operate to move the hip as separate groups. They also work together to actively provide stability and position the bones of the joint so that the head of your femur doesn't press into the passive structures (like the labrum, cartilage, or ligaments) around your hip joint.

KEY POINT:
Dealing with Sciatic Nerve Pain

Piriformis Syndrome is a term commonly used to describe nerve pain resulting from irritation or compression of the sciatic nerve by the piriformis. Sometimes, you will hear this phenomenon also referred to as a form of sciatica. Whatever you call it, it's pretty annoying.

Your sciatic nerves are the largest nerves in your body. These nerves begin in your lower spine and run through your hips and thighs, then branch off to become smaller nerves that run through your lower legs and into your feet. Sciatica is pain that radiates along the sciatic nerve.

For most of us, the sciatic nerve runs directly underneath the piriformis. However, in some people the sciatic nerve runs partially or completely through the center of the piriformis. Additionally, in rare cases, it can run right over the top of the piriformis—another indication that while we humans are all the same species, there can be many different variations in our anatomy that make us all very unique.

When the piriformis is pressing on or irritating the sciatic nerve, often people are told to stretch their piriformis in an attempt to release the tension that is impinging on the nerve. However, stretching your piriformis pulls the muscle taut and puts tension on it, which can further irritate the nerve. So the key is to find a mild stretch that you can sustain without further aggravating the nerve.

While your piriformis may be irritating or compressing your sciatic nerve giving rise to sciatic nerve pain, the pain also can be the result of compression of the nerve at your spine. Don't make assumptions about its origin. Instead, consult your medical professional if you experience sciatic nerve pain in order to determine the true origin and take appropriate action to minimize and manage the pain.

The Knee Joint

Your knee joint is a complex structure that consists of three bones—the bottom part of your femur, the top part of your tibia (the big shinbone), and your patella (the kneecap). Your femur and tibia form the top and bottom of this hinge-like structure, with the flat top of your tibia forming the base of the hinge and the rounded knobs of the lower part of your femur forming the top of the hinge. Your patella is housed inside the connective tissue that crosses over the joint from your rectus femoris to your shinbone. The patella sits in a groove at the front of the femur, gliding over the hinge of the joint as the joint moves. Your patella provides a layer of bony protection to the front of the joint and the passive joint structures underneath, but it also provides additional friction protection to the patellar tendon itself which moves over the bones numerous times every day.

On top of the bones are two types of cartilage. First, you have the thin, smooth, and slippery articular cartilage that lines the surface of the bones so they can glide over each other. You also have two thick pads of cartilage called menisci—or separately called a meniscus. These pads sit on top of the tibia, help to stabilize the knee joint, and act as shock-absorbing cushions in the space where your femur and your tibia come together.

Four strong ligaments hold the bones of your knee together and keep them from moving out of alignment with each other. You have two collateral ligaments (medial collateral ligament or MCL and lateral collateral ligament or LCL) which prevent your knee from moving side to side and two cruciate ligaments (anterior cruciate ligament or ACL and posterior cruciate ligament or PCL) which prevent the forward and backward movement of the bones over each other. These ligaments act like strong ropes that connect and hold the bones in position in relation to each other.

Most of the responsibility for stability of your knee joint rests with this sophisticated family of ligaments, which is one of the reasons why knee injuries—particularly those caused by collision—tend to be things that haunt you for the rest of your life. The ligaments, once stretched, never really go back to the way they were, which means that they lose some of their capacity to effectively stabilize and support the joint. If they get stretched too far, they can tear away from the bone.

Two more structures contribute greatly to the stability of your knee joint: (1) the patellar ligament, sometimes called the patellar tendon, that connects your kneecap to your shin bone and (2) the iliotibial (IT) band, a thickening of the fascia that wraps around your thigh muscles and runs from your outer hip down to your outer knee.

KNEE MOVEMENTS

Despite the complexity of the joint structure itself, compared to the hip movements we've investigated, the movements of your knee will seem much simpler. A healthy knee can move two ways:

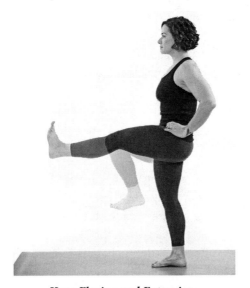

Knee Flexion and Extension.

- Knee Flexion: occurs when you bend your knee
- Knee Extension: occurs when you straighten your knee

The hinge design of the knee gives it far less movement potential than the ball and socket configuration of the hip joint and many of the other major joints covered in this book.

The Knee Muscles

While most of the stability for the knee comes from the ligaments that bind the bones of your knee joint together, the muscles in your upper and lower leg that cross the knee joint provide some additional stability.

From the upper thigh, there are two groups of muscles that move and help stabilize your knees:

- Quadriceps: four muscles that cover the front of your thigh and attach to the top of your kneecap and down to the front of your shinbone via the patellar ligament. This group is responsible for knee extension.
- Hamstrings: three muscles at the back of your thigh that cross over your knee joint to attach to your tibia and fibula (your two shinbones). These muscles work together to flex your knee.

As you may recall from the previous chapter, the gastrocnemius muscle in your lower leg also crosses your knee and assists your hamstrings with knee flexion.

Additionally, the lateral stabilizers of your hip also play a key role in the positioning of your knee, particularly while running.

KEY POINT: *The IT Band*

The IT band is something most runners have heard a lot about. Mostly, because it's a common area of pain among distance runners. It's also probably one of the most misunderstood tissues in the body. There is so much misinformation spread about the IT band, what it does, and what you should do when you feel that telltale pain at the outer part of your knee every time you bend your knee.

The muscles of your thigh are all encased in a wrapper of fascia called the fascia latae, the fascia of the side. There is a strip that runs down your outer thigh which is significantly thicker and more fibrous than the rest of the wrapper—this is your IT band. In other words, your IT band is not a separate structure. It's not really a band that has edges that separate it from the structures around it. It's a thickening of the fascia that runs from your outer hip down to your outer knee.

This thickening is there in order to provide more lateral support and stability for your hip and knee joints and to create cohesion between them. Because its job is to add stability that spans two major weight-bearing joints, you need it to be strong and taut. By design, there is very little elastin in your IT band, which means it has very little capacity to stretch—and you really don't want it to. It's also not a muscle with the ability to contract, so it could not be supportive if it were loose and stretchy.

What's really going on here, then, and how do you fix it?

It is common for the tissues that attach to the IT band near the outer hip to become tight, which creates the feeling of tension in the IT band. It is also possible that one of your quadriceps muscles—specifically vastus lateralis at the outer thigh—can adhere to the IT band. This tends to occur in bodies where there is significant repetitive movement of the IT band sliding over the muscle layer beneath it, an action that happens in running. This repetitive motion can create an area of high friction, resulting in the body producing and laying down an abundance of collagen fibers between these layers of tissue. These collagen fibers may ultimately form cross-links between the layers of tissue, binding them together. This can make your IT band feel "tight" and restricted as well. In some situations, IT band pain can be related to weakness or inactivity in the lateral stabilizer muscles in the hip.

For years, a common form of "treatment" for pain associated with the IT band has been to roll the whole length of the IT band with a foam roller. And over the years, I've seen many people take a very aggressive approach to this, many of them believing that the pain of rolling on their IT band means they need to roll more and with greater pressure. This approach of punishing the IT band has not produced positive long-term results in any of the athletes I've worked with. Nor do I think this is an appropriate attitude to take toward any of the tissues in your body that work so hard to support you. Instead, you'd be better served by investigating the underlying reasons why your IT band feels tight—many of these are covered by the work in this book.

A number of pain receptors all around your IT band are very intentionally warning you to stay away. Please do your IT band a favor and stop punishing it by rolling around aimlessly on your foam roller. We can do better than this, I promise.

Give the mobility and myofascial release work in this chapter a try—specifically the Low Lunge Side Bend, self-myofascial release work prescribed for your tensor fascia latae and your outer quads, and the Clamshells exercise—to target the specific areas that may be causing your IT band to feel tight. You'll probably see that you get better results with a lot less punishment on your poor IT band, which is trying its best to hold you together with every step you take.

Common Issues Among Runners

Most of the injuries associated with the hip in runners are related to one or a combination of two things.

- Weakness or inactivity in the lateral stabilizers resulting in too much movement through the lower back, hips, and/or the knee;
- Imbalances in the relative strength, activation, and range of motion between the muscles that work in opposition with each other to move the hip joint.

Let's examine these separately.

Most of our lives are oriented forward, as is the sport of running. But your body was meant to move in many different planes of motion, and as a result you have 360 degrees of muscles that wrap around your hips and support you. When you neglect these other planes of motion and move your limbs only forward and backward, you don't make use of certain muscles, so they go dormant. Think of it as them falling out of the communication loop when they don't get called upon to activate. This is a common issue with the lateral stabilizers. When you forget to train these muscles to activate and keep your hips level, with every step you take in your running stride one hip dips below the level of the other, causing issues from lower back pain to knee pain.

If you spend large portions of your day sitting in hip flexion, the odds are that the tissues at the front of your hips are tight. Remember that the muscles that create movement in the hips are also working together to dynamically position the bones and stabilize the joint. When the muscles on one side of the joint are allowed to pull more on the bones, there is a tendency for the head of the femur to shift in the socket and start pushing into the cartilage and labrum. When you add the repeated impact of running to that scenario, you've got a solid recipe for pain and joint degeneration.

Additionally, habits build up in the tissues of your body. The repeated postures and movements you make every day—whether consciously or not—have the potential to create or exacerbate muscular imbalances not only in terms of tissue tension and mobility but also in terms of strength. A balanced running stride requires balanced strength among the muscles that work cooperatively through every stage of the gait cycle to propel you forward. Often runners develop dominance in one muscle group (typically the hip flexors and quadriceps) over the opposing muscle group (in this case, the gluteus maximus and hamstrings). This can lead to an overreliance on certain muscles during the gait cycle, which is not only inefficient but can also lead to movement compensations and ultimately overuse injuries.

Now let's look specifically at the knee. Since running tends not to be a collision sport (at least not the way I do it), many of the knee injuries that occur in sports with collision potential are not present in the sport of running, though having sustained a previous traumatic injury to the ligaments or cartilage in your knee may make running painful or problematic for you. Aside from preexisting knee injuries, most knee problems in runners are inflammation issues. Generally, these occur from straining the connective tissues by doing too much, too soon or from kneecap tracking issues related to muscular imbalances in the muscles that move the knee through its range of motion.

How to Fix It

In order to keep your hips and knees healthy and happy and logging a lifetime of miles, you have to (1) preserve the ability of your hips to move well in all directions; (2) spend a little more time in positions that allow tighter or overused tissues to be in a lengthened position; (3) apply some mild to moderate compression to promote circulation and facilitate better glide between the layers of tissue in high friction areas; and (4) train the muscles of your hips and thighs to be balanced, functional, and strong to better support an efficient and powerful running stride.

The Movement Practices

Mobilize and Release Your Hips and Upper Legs

Since many of us already spend sufficient time in hip flexion, we'll work to mobilize the tissues that flex the hip as well as the surrounding tissues that are typically in a shortened position when running and sitting.

EQUIPMENT/PROPS NEEDED: two yoga blocks, a bolster, and a blanket.

Supported Bridge with Long Reach

Grab a yoga block and lie on your back with your knees bent and feet flat on the floor. Press your feet into the floor to lift your hips. Place the block on either its lowest height or middle height under the back of your

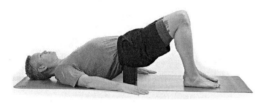

Supported Bridge.

pelvis (below your lower back) and set your hips on the block. Try to relax your lower back and as you stay in this position and breathe, think about the bones of your lower back being heavy and softening down toward the floor. If this feels too intense on your lower back, drop the block down a level or use a rolled up blanket under your hips instead. Stay for a few breaths.

From the Supported Bridge position (see above), extend your right leg long and set your right heel on the floor. Then, extend your left leg out as well. Shake your feet a little from side to side so they relax. Continue to let your lower back relax and get heavier toward the floor. If it feels comfortable, take your arms up by your head and let them rest on the floor but don't let your low back arch to where you feel compression or pinching in your lumbar spine. Stay for 1–2

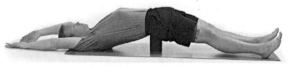

Long Reach Variation.

minutes. Then lift your hips, remove the block, and drop your knees from side to side a few times.

BLOCK PSOAS STRETCH

From the Supported Bridge position (see above), hug your left knee into your chest and extend your right leg long with your right heel resting on the floor. With a small bend in your right knee, as you inhale, press your right heel down into the floor and stretch it away from your head. As you exhale, draw your left knee in a little closer. Your legs should feel active and engaged but relax your hips and lower back. Stay for 5 breaths and then switch sides.

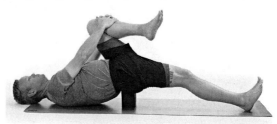

Block Psoas Stretch.

SUPPORTED SADDLE

Set a yoga block up at its middle or highest height at the back of your mat as shown below. Lay a bolster over both blocks so it forms a ramp and place a folded blanket at the far end of the bolster to use as a pillow. Another option if you need to be up higher with more support is to use the two block setup shown on page 115. Come into all fours on your hands and knees with your toes right beside the edges of your bolster. Bring your toes together and sit back so that your hips are resting over your heels. If the tops of your feet or ankles are not happy here, roll up a blanket or towel and place it under you. Keep your feet together with your hips on top of your heels and then separate your knees. Lower yourself back onto the bolster and rest your hands somewhere comfortable. Stay here for 5 minutes. When you come back up, go forward into all fours, tuck your toes under, and take your heels from side to side to shake out your legs.

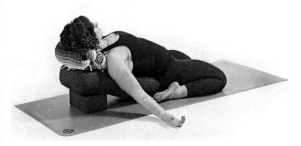

Supported Saddle.

SUPPORTED STRADDLE

Sit up tall with your legs comfortably wide and relatively straight. As you start to lean forward slightly, think about your ASIS points tipping forward toward the floor—as if you were lightly arching your lower back.

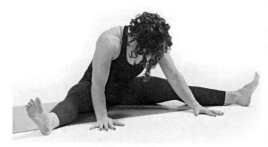

Supported Straddle.

Place your hands on the floor in front of you. Once your shoulders have come forward of your hips, to round your spine and tuck your chin into your chest as you lean into the support of your arms and relax. Stay here for 10 or more breaths. You can also sit up on a folded blanket to help encourage your pelvis to tilt forward or place your hands on the floor behind your hips and lean back into them.

BUTTERFLY STRETCH

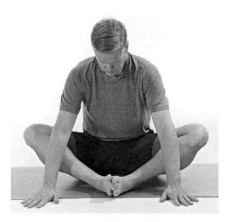

Butterfly Stretch.

Sit up tall and bring the soles of your feet together and let your knees fall open and out to the sides. Your feet should be comfortably close to your hips—don't force them. Grab on to your ankles or your feet and as you inhale, sit up to your full height. Maintain the height in your spine as you exhale and lean forward, leading with your chest. Once your shoulders have come forward of your hips, round your spine and tuck your chin into your chest. If you would like more support, it's helpful to place your hands on the floor beside your feet, straighten but don't lock your elbows, and lean into the support of your arms. Do not force or press your thighs down; instead, think about the tops of your thighbones softening down into the floor. Stay here for 10 or more breaths.

LOW LUNGE STRETCH

From hands and knees, step your right foot forward between your hands. Keep your left knee on the floor, left toes tucked or untucked, whichever you prefer. Place both your hands on your right thigh and come up into a low lunge. As you inhale, press your hands into your thigh and curl your low belly up and away from your front thigh as you think about lifting the front rim of your pelvis upward. Maintain the slight posterior tilt in your pelvis as you exhale and lower your hips a little toward the floor—they won't go far without losing the tilt.

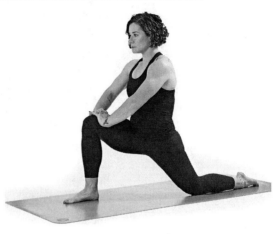

Low Lunge Stretch.

Repeat 2 more times. Inhale to curl your spine back and lift the front rim of your pelvis, exhale to lower your hips. Then, switch sides.

Low Lunge Side Bend

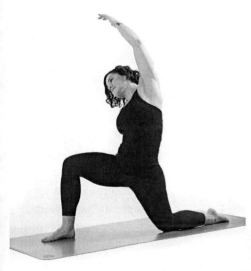

Low Lunge Side Bend.

From hands and knees, step your right foot forward between your hands. Keep your left knee on the floor, left toes tucked or untucked, whichever you prefer. Come up into a low lunge. Place your right hand on your right hip and reach up with your left arm. Think about lifting the front rim of your pelvis upward and maintain this position of your pelvis as you lean to your right. Draw your front ribs back so it's a side bend rather than a back bend. Hold for 3–5 breaths and switch sides.

Bound Twisted Low Lunge

From hands and knees, step your right foot forward between your hands. Keep your left knee and left hand on the floor as you rotate your torso toward your right thigh and place your right hand on your right thigh. You can stay in this position or reach back with your right hand, bend your left knee to lift your left foot up, and grab your left foot with your right hand. Gently press your left thigh just above your knee into the floor as you lift your low belly up and away from the floor. Hold for 5 breaths and switch sides.

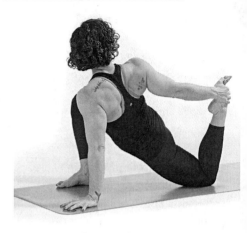

Bound Twisted Low Lunge.

Reclined Figure 4 Stretch

Lie on your back with your feet flat on the floor and your knees bent. Cross your left ankle over your right thigh just above your right knee. Lift your right foot up and bring your legs toward your chest. Grab the back of your right thigh with your hands and relax your head and shoulders on the floor. Your tailbone will lift away from the floor a little—it's not a bad thing, but try to minimize it. Stay here for 5–8 breaths and then switch sides.

NOTE: If you experience any sharp or radiating nerve pain through the back of your hip or down your leg while in this stretch, ease up and be more gentle—perhaps even do this stretch with your legs up a wall.

As we discussed earlier in this chapter, sciatic nerve pain can be amplified by stretching or otherwise pulling your piriformis taut in positions such as this. Find a position where the stretch is gentle enough to not aggravate the nerve.

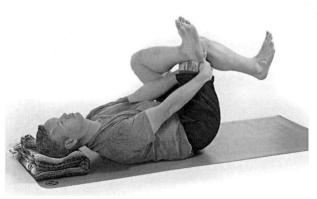

Reclined Figure 4 Stretch.

RECLINED CROSS-LEGGED STRETCH

Lie on your back with your feet flat on the floor and your knees bent. Cross your right thigh over your left thigh above your knee and bring your thighs toward your chest. Grab on to opposite knees, shins, or ankles with your hands and relax your head and shoulders on the floor. Your tailbone will lift away from the floor a little—try to mini-

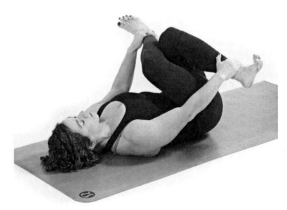

Reclined Cross-Legged Stretch.

mize it and press your tailbone down. Use your arms to gently pull your shins away from the midline of your body. Stay here for 5–8 breaths and then switch sides.

SIDE-LYING QUAD STRETCH

Lie on your right side with your hips and legs stacked. Rest your head on your right upper arm or hold your head in your hand. Bend your left knee and reach back with your left hand to grab your left foot or ankle. Press your hips slightly forward and gently lift the front rim of your pelvis up in the direction in of your ribs. Stay for 5–10 breaths and then switch sides.

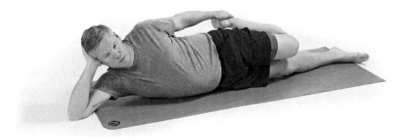

Side-Lying Quad Stretch.

LEGS UP THE WALL

Sit with your right side against the wall. Swing your legs up onto the wall and lower your shoulders and head onto the floor. Position your hips as close to the wall as is comfortable for your legs and lower back. If it feels more comfortable for you, you can place a folded blanket under the back of your hips (below your lower back). Stay for 5 minutes or more.

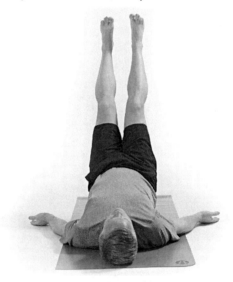

Legs Up the Wall.

Roll and Release Your Hips

In this section, we'll apply some gentle compression to stimulate circulation to and reoxygenation of these tissues that have a tendency to be tense due to postural and movement habits. We'll also work on the areas that tend to be less active in runners and people who sit a lot, and we'll zero in on one of the high friction zones in runners where collagen fibers tend to adhere the layers of tissue together creating the feeling of tension on the IT band.

You might notice that the iliopsoas is not listed below. Not to worry, we'll hit that in the next chapter when we deal with the lumbar spine and core.

IMPORTANT NOTE: There are many delicate structures that run through your hips and inner thighs particularly near the groin area such as large nerves and arteries. Steer clear of anything that feels painful, sharp, or radiates out into other areas of your body. We're looking for sensation that is dull and achy but that you can still relax and soften into. If at any point, you start to feel tingling or numbness, move off the spot you're on and work on surrounding tissues that do not cause altered or loss of sensation.

EQUIPMENT/PROPS NEEDED: a yoga block and a myofascial ball.

MIDDLE QUADS

From hands and knees, bring your right knee forward toward your right wrist and rest your right shin and foot on the floor with your right knee bent. Lower yourself down to your elbows and extend your left leg straight back from your left hip. Place a myofascial ball directly above your left knee so that the bottom of the ball is touching the

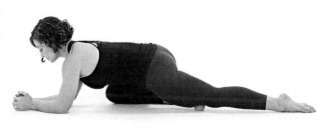

top edge of your kneecap. You can keep your left leg extended or you can slowly bend and straighten your left knee as you put some gentle pressure just above your

Middle Quads https://youtu.be/fPXhDZNIoNs

left kneecap. Spend about 20 seconds or so on that spot. If you were moving your left leg, pause and be still for a breath before moving on.

Now, move the ball about an inch or two up the center of your left thigh and repeat. You can keep your left leg extended and work to relax your left thigh as you breathe or slowly bend and straighten your leg. Spend about 20 seconds or so on that spot. If you were moving your left leg, remember to pause and be still for a breath before moving on.

Then, move the ball up another inch so that you are about one-third of the way up your left thigh. Be still or bend and straighten your left leg. Try to keep your left thigh heavy either way.

After 20 seconds or so, move the ball up so it's about half way or just a little above halfway up your left thigh and repeat the process. Remain still and breathe as you relax into it or bend and straighten your leg. Stay here for about 20 seconds. Repeat on your right leg.

OUTER QUADS

This technique is similar in set-up to the middle quads release work described above, but instead of working up the front of your thigh, we'll be just slightly toward the outer edge of the top of your thigh with your body angled a bit as pictured. However, it's important to note that this version is intended to work on the high friction area where the IT band tends to get adhered to the outer quads muscle right underneath it. Because of that, this version tends to feel more intense.

Begin in the same position as shown above in the middle quads release work, except for this variation you'll place a myofascial ball directly above the outer corner of your left kneecap and angle your torso toward the

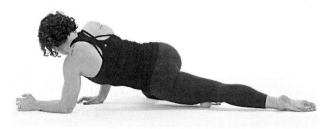

right. For this work, the ball is not on the front of your thigh and not on the side of your thigh—it's somewhere in between the front and outside of your left thigh. Once you get

Outer Quads https://youtu.be/Ye8YRWCVXlo

into position, perform the same steps as detailed above, slowly moving up your outer thigh, applying gentle compression and being still or bending and straightening your left leg. Once you've gotten about two-thirds of the way up your left thigh, switch sides.

Gluteus Medius

Lie on your back with your knees bent and feet flat on the floor. Place a myofascial ball under the back of your right hip toward the top outer portion of the fleshy part of your glutes—basically, where your right back pocket would be in a pair of fitted jeans. Extend your right leg and roll more of your weigh onto your right hip as you support yourself on your right forearm. Stay in the outer, upper area of your glutes. When you find a tender spot, be still, breathe, and try to soften into it as you relax your whole right leg as much as possible. Stay for 20–30 seconds and then move around a little bit

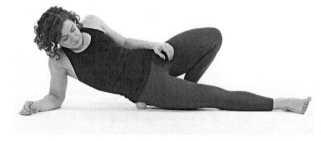

Gluteus Medius https://youtu.be/rQoq2SjPUcw

in that area and find another tender spot where you can stay for a few breaths. Remove the ball and lie flat on your back for a few moments to feel the effects of working on this area. Then, repeat on your left leg.

TENSOR FASCIA LATAE

Lie on your left side with your hips stacked and your legs extended. Prop yourself up on your left forearm, bend your right knee and place it on the floor in front of you, and angle your torso slightly downward. With your finger, locate the bony landmark of your ASIS point on the front of your left hip. Place a my-ofascial ball just to

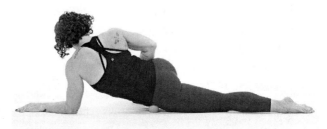

Tensor Fascia Latae https://youtu.be/dwDHDPfcDBQ

the left of this landmark and about level with your pubic bone. You're aiming to put the ball somewhere between the front and outer portions of your left hip where your front pocket would be. Wiggle around a little in that area until you find a tender spot then hold still and breathe as you try to relax into it. Stay for 20–30 seconds. Then, move the ball around a little to find another tender spot where you can stay for a few breaths. Remove the ball and lie flat on your back for a few moments to notice any difference in sensation from one side versus the other. Then, repeat on your right leg.

PIRIFORMIS

Lie on your back with your knees bent and feet flat on the floor. Place a myofascial ball under the back of your left hip just below the center of the fleshy part of your glutes. Cross your left ankle over your right thigh and lean a little over toward your left hip. Wiggle around slowly and carefully until you find a tender spot where you

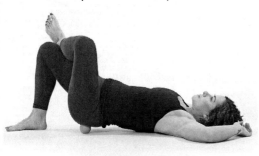

Piriformis https://youtu.be/bAiKu9i61W8

can stay, relax, and breathe for 20–30 seconds. Avoid anything sharp, radiating, or painful here—you are very close to one of your sciatic nerves. When you're done on this side, remove the ball and lie flat on your back for a few moments to feel the effects of this release work. Then, repeat on your right hip.

ADDUCTORS

Lie on your right side with your hips stacked and your legs extended. Prop your head up in your right hand and bend your left knee and rest it on a block at hip level. Begin with the block close to your left knee and place a myofascial ball at the center of your inner left thigh just above the bony spot there. For all the trigger points in this work, we'll be working up the inner thigh as if we're following an imaginary line along the inseam

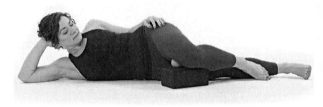

Adductors https://youtu.be/FYQwSu6QrJA

of your pants. Once you get into this first position close to your knee, let your left leg be heavy and relaxed. You can either remain still and let the ball sink into the tissues there or slowly bend and straighten your left knee. Spend a few breaths on that spot. If you were moving your left leg, pause and be still for a breath before moving on.

Now, move the ball about an inch or two up that imaginary inseam and repeat. You have the options to remain still here or slowly bend and straighten your leg. Spend a few breaths on that spot. If you were moving your left leg, remember to pause and be still for a breath before moving on.

Then, move the ball up another inch so that you are about one-third of the way up your inner left thigh. Be still or bend and straighten your left leg. Stay here for a few breaths.

Roll onto your back and take a few rounds of breath to notice any difference in sensation between your right and left sides. Roll onto your left side and repeat on your right leg.

Balance and Strengthen Your Hips

In this section, we'll work on developing more strength and activation in the muscles that have a tendency to be a little more dormant than the larger and more dominant muscles around the hip. We'll fire up your posterior chain (the muscles on the back of your hips and thighs) so that they're ready to power your running stride.

Additionally, since most of the work in this chapter is unilateral (meaning one leg is working at a time) you'll have the opportunity to see if there are imbalances in the strength and stability of one leg versus your other leg. But don't get too bent out of shape if you find that to be the case. Most of us have discrepancies between the two sides of our bodies, some of which are the result of habits and others are related more to the inherent asymmetry of our anatomy (for example, your heart is on the left side of your chest and your liver is on the right side of your torso). Unless it's contributing to injuries or discomfort, it's worth knowing and attempting to minimize the extent of such discrepancies, but it's not worth making a big deal of it.

Be mindful as you work through these exercises that the position of your hips has an effect on your lower back and vice versa. None of this work should cause you lower back pain or discomfort. If you do experience lower back pain while doing these exercises, or immediately after, it's likely that you are not properly supporting your spine enough during that movement. It's a good habit to get into to learn to engage your core in a way that is more supportive of your lower back. You can find lots of ways to do that in the next chapter, which I encourage you to read in conjunction with this chapter, as these two areas are intimately connected.

EQUIPMENT/PROPS NEEDED: slider disc (or kitchen towel), a yoga block, some mini bands, and a long resistance band.

BANDED GLUTE BRIDGES

Place a mini band around your upper shins or just above your knees and lie on your back with your knees bent and your feet flat on the floor. Press into your feet to lift your hips up as you press your legs out into the band to keep them from caving inward. Once your knees, hips, and shoulders form a straight line, gently draw your pubic bone up toward your lower ribs to

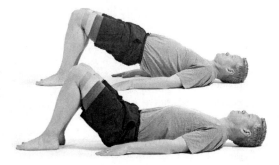

Banded Glute Bridges.

engage your core. Keep your tailbone lengthening away from your head and focus on creating a moderate muscular contraction in the lower fibers of your gluteus maximus (near your sit bones) but don't vigorously clench them. Slowly lower back down without letting the band pull your knees in and repeat. Perform 3–5 sets of 6 slow reps per side.

CLAMSHELLS

Place a mini band around both of your legs just below your knees and lie on your left side with your hips, knees, and ankles stacked. Bend your knees and bring them slightly in front of your torso. Keep your heels together but lift your right knee up and away from your right knee as high as you can without moving your pelvis or leaning back with your hips or torso—it's not about how far your knee moves, it's about quality and stability. Be

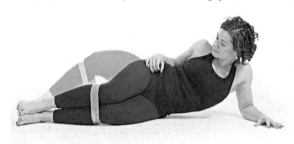

Clamshells https://youtu.be/wmxipFZxo50

sure that your hips stay stacked over each other. Pause at the top for a moment and then return to the starting position and repeat. Perform 3–5 sets of 10 reps per side.

SUPINE BAND PULLS

Place a mini band around your feet and lie on your back. Place your hands on your lower ribs, and gently draw them back. Gently press your lower back toward the floor and use your core to maintain that position as you bend your left knee and draw it toward your chest against the resistance of the mini band. Slowly and with control, return your left leg to the starting position and repeat. Perform 3–5 sets of 10 reps per side.

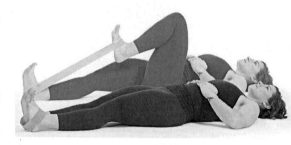

Supine Band Pulls.

SINGLE LEG GLUTE BRIDGES

Lie on your back with your knees bent and your feet flat on the floor. Extend your arms upward so that your palms face each other and your hands are directly over your shoulders. Press your upper back into the floor for stability. Gently press your entire lower back into the floor. Lift your left leg up so that your left knee is directly over your left hip with your left

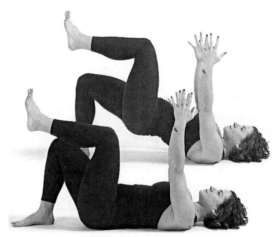

Single Leg Glute Bridges.

shin parallel to the floor. Press into your right foot to lift your hips up. Keep your hips level throughout the movement and don't let your lower back arch as you lift and lower. Perform 8–10 reps per side.

BOAT HOLD WITH TOE TAPS

Sit with your knees bent and feet flat on the floor. Place your hands behind your thighs and lean your torso back just enough that you can lift your feet up with your shins parallel to the floor. Lengthen your spine so that your torso is stretched to its full height and broaden through your

chest. If this is easy for you, release your hands from your thighs and reach forward with your fingers. Hold this position for 30 seconds but do not let your torso slouch or your lower back sink and round. Stay lifted through your torso and chest. If the 30-second hold is easy for you, you can add greater

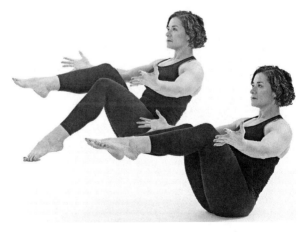

Boat Hold with Toe Taps.

challenge by alternating lowering and tapping one foot at a time to the floor. Move slowly and keep your spine long. If performing toe taps, do 20 taps (10 per side) alternating sides. Perform 3–5 sets of the hold or toe taps.

HAMSTRING SLIDES

Lie on your back with your knees bent and your feet flat on the floor. Place a slider disc under your left foot (or if you're on a hard surface you can use a kitchen towel instead). Press into both of your feet to lift your hips up and engage your core by gently drawing your pubic bone up toward your lower ribs so your lower back doesn't arch. Keep your right foot where it is and your hips level

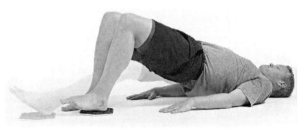

Hamstring Slides.

as you slowly (over 3–5 seconds) slide your left foot along the floor to straighten your left leg. Once your leg is fully extended, lower your hips to the floor with control and draw your left leg back to meet your right and repeat. Perform 3–5 sets of 6 slow reps per side.

ADDUCTOR BAND PULLS

Anchor a long resistance band low, close to floor level. Place the other end of the band on your right foot and step far enough away from the anchor point that you've taken up the slack and there's some mild tension on the band. Stand up tall with your feet under your hips. Draw your right foot toward the

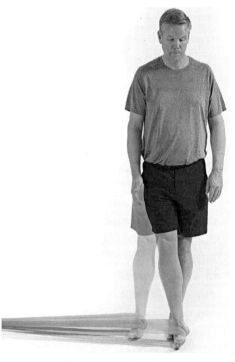

Adductor Band Pulls.

midline of your body and in front of your left leg. Pause there for a second and then slowly return your right foot to the starting position and repeat. Perform 3–5 sets of 10 reps per side.

Foot Banded Lateral Walks

Place a mini band around the balls of both of your feet. Bend your knees slightly to come into a quarter-squat position with your second and third toes pointing straight ahead and your knees directly over your toes. Place your hands on your hips and pick your left foot up and step it to the left. Then step your right foot toward your left foot. Try not to shift your hips with each step and don't let your toes or knees turn inward or outward—keep them both pointed straight ahead. Then repeat by stepping again to the left with your left foot, followed by your right foot. Perform 3–5 sets of 10 steps per side.

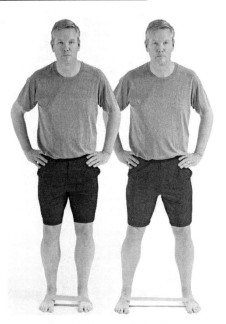

Foot Banded Lateral Walks.

Heel Dips

Stand with your feet on a step or block with your hands on your hips. Lift your right foot up and move it slightly in front of the step. Keep your hips level and your left knee tracking in line with your second and third toes as you bend your left knee far enough to tap your right heel to the floor just in front of you. Be sure that your left knee is not caving inward. Press into your left foot to straighten

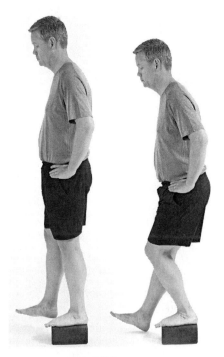

Heel Dips.

your left leg and return to standing with your right foot hovering off the floor. Perform 3–5 sets of 10 reps per leg.

Slider Side Lunges

Stand tall, feet under your hips, with your right foot on a slider disc and your left foot on the floor. Slide the disc out to your right side as you bend your left knee and press your hips back. Aim to get your left thigh parallel to the ground (or as close as comfortably possible) and keep your left knee tracking in the same direction as your second and third toes—don't let

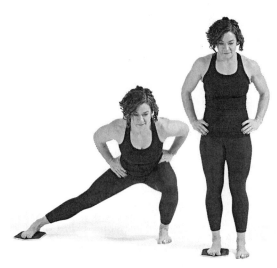

Slider Side Lunges.

your knee drift inward or outward. Carefully return to standing by sliding your right foot back to the starting position and repeat. Perform 3–5 sets of 10 reps per side.

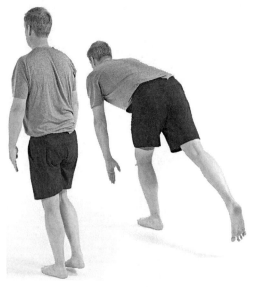

Single Leg Deadlift.

Single Leg Deadlift

Stand tall with your feet hip-width distance apart, toes pointed straight ahead. Lift your right foot to hover just above the floor. Press your hips back and reach your right leg behind you as you hinge from your hips, bend your left knee slightly, and reach toward the floor with your hands. Be sure to keep your hips square to the floor and level with each other. Keep your left shin upright and perpendicular to the floor and your right leg active and reaching straight back so that it doesn't cross the midline of your body or swing out to the left side. Don't round your shoulders forward as you lower down and keep your core engaged (think pubic bone and low ribs gently drawing toward each other). To return to standing, press your whole left foot (ball and heel) into the floor as you bring your hips forward and rise to stand. Perform 3–5 sets of 10 reps per side.

Notes on Running Form

Remember, the tissues in your body adapt and conform to the things you do most often. So if you're like me (and many other runners), you need to be aware of how these patterns can affect your running form and running stride. Additionally, you need to be proactive in your approach to minimizing any range of motion or strength imbalances that your lifestyle may be having on your running posture. The work described in this chapter will certainly help you get there if you practice consistently.

It's important that you also practice maintaining a neutral pelvic positioning while running. This will enable you to access the strength and power of your legs as well as move all the joints of your lower body through a full range of motion. The positioning of your hips in conjunction with the movement of your legs can make all the difference between having a fluid running stride and wasting energy.

Here are some things to keep in mind when you're running to ensure that you're practicing a running posture that will support you well for years to come.

- **Do keep your hip bones pointing forward.** Remember the ASIS points we talked about in this chapter? Keep them pointed straight ahead. This is especially important if you know that you already tend to tilt your pelvis anteriorly. When runners get tired, often those ASIS points start to tilt downward, putting more pressure on the lower back. Think of the structure of your pelvis as being like a bowl full of marbles and your goal is to not lose any of those marbles by tipping the bowl too far forward.
- **Do keep your hip bones level.** In addition to keeping them pointed straight ahead, you want your ASIS points to remain

pretty level. This is a key indication that your pelvic stabilizers are working well for you.

- **Don't exaggerate your knee lift.** Efficient endurance running requires a slight knee lift as your knee comes forward—but you don't want to exaggerate it similar to the way you would if you were sprinting.

- **Do turn your legs over quickly.** Your stride should be fairly short and compact, with your lower leg not extending or reaching out in front of you. Minimize the amount of time that your feet are on the ground.

- **Don't bounce.** To help control any bouncing, be sure that your feet land underneath your body, not out in front of you. The more energy you put into going up, the less you have to go forward.

Part 3: Core and Lower Back

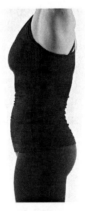

Support yourself better.

Lower back pain isn't unique to runners. But it certainly can make running pretty miserable. Lower back pain can leave you with many questions, wondering if you're injured or just achy ... and why? You don't have to be injured to experience lower back pain. And as positive as that sounds on the surface, it's also the thing that makes dealing with lower back pain incredibly frustrating. Sometimes there just isn't anything going on there that can be classified as an injury in the traditional sense.

That's not to say that you can't injure your lower back—you certainly can. Several common injuries can occur in the lumbar spine, the most common being disc issues like bulges and herniations. Alignment of this sophisticated column of bones and the spinal cord they protect is critical, and there is potential for the structure to shift through a number of scenarios that can be extraordinarily painful. However, it is possible to have disc issues and no lower back pain. It is also possible to have pain in your lower back and not have any structural damage or dysfunction. Crazy, right?

It often begins as a deep, achy feeling in your lower back. This pain is typically symmetrical and centered so it feels like it's literally in the bones of your lumbar spine. It's a feeling that no amount of massage or stretching seems to remedy for long. In fact, the only thing that seems to help is changing positions and avoiding certain postures—like rounding or arching your lower back.

For runners, this pain may or may not have started as a result of running, but it most certainly can affect their ability to run comfortably. Such pain is one of the most common issues I see in newer runners and those returning to the sport from breaks. Sadly, many of these individuals don't continue running because they believe that running is "bad" for their backs. But it's generally something that my durability training protocol can provide relief from.

The primary function of your core during running is to stabilize your spine and minimize the amount of localized bending and twisting in your lumbar spine. Your core is designed to provide 360 degrees of support from the bottom of your ribs to the top of your pelvis as well as precise adjustments in order to maintain a neutral position for your spine. In order to keep your spine healthy and happy, you need to train the core muscles in a way that maximizes their potential to support you well.

Anatomy and Physiology Basics

The Spine

In this chapter, we'll be dealing primarily with the lumbar spine and its relationship to the muscles of the core. But it's useful to take a look at the spine as a unit, since it's the skeletal scaffolding that forms the framework of your trunk from skull to pelvis.

Your spine is made up of 24 individual bones called vertebrae; of the discs situated between each of these bones; of your sacrum, which joins your spine to the back of your pelvis; and your coccyx or, as it's more commonly known, your tailbone.

The vertebrae are divided into three sections based on where they are located in relation to your rib cage.

- The cervical spine: the first seven vertebrae starting at the base of your skull, down through your neck to just above your rib cage—referred individually as C-1 through C-7 (numbered from top to bottom).

- The thoracic spine: the middle 12 vertebrae starting at your first ribs at the base of your neck and continuing down your spine to the 12th rib at the bottom of your rib cage—referred individually as T-1 through T-12 (top to bottom).
- The lumbar spine: the last five vertebrae starting from just below your last ribs down to your sacrum—referred individually as L-1 through L-5 (top to bottom).

In between each set of vertebrae that form this long chainlike structure of your spine are squishy discs that serve a couple of critical functions. First, they give your spine the ability to articulate so you can move in the very interesting and somewhat snakelike way you can through your spine and torso. These discs also provide shock absorption and force distribution. As people who enjoy a sport that involves as much impact as running does, we should all be thankful for this attribute.

If you were to look at a model of a human spine, you'd see that not all vertebrae look the same. Most notably, the size of the vertebrae get bigger the further down the spine you go. This phenomenon falls in line with the weight-bearing demands placed on each section of the spine. Consider how much less weight the vertebrae in your neck have to support versus the vertebrae in your lower back.

Each level of your spine has three weight-bearing points of contact. The vertebral bodies and discs that separate them form one point of contact at the front of your spinal column. At the back of your spine, on either side of the vertebral bodies, are a pair of little bony knobs that fit together with the vertebrae above and below them. These are called facet joints. Facet joints are lined with cartilage and have just enough space between them to allow for your spine's trademark mobility while also creating a backstop to large movements and providing the much-needed stability to the structure of your spine.

The way that you position your spine determines the distribution of weight among those weight-bearing points of the spine. When you run or even when you sit, there is potential for the lower back to move out of its neutral position—where the weight is evenly distributed among the three points of contact—and into a position where more of the load is shifted onto either (1) the discs at the front of your spine or (2) the two facet joints at the back of the spine. This concept has some really important implications for our investigation of injury and pain later in this chapter.

Your spine houses and protects your spinal cord. Proper alignment of all the pieces ensures the preservation of the small openings between each of your vertebrae where your spinal nerves branch off of your spinal cord and exit your spinal column. Any shifting of the pieces or misalignments can pinch or damage these nerves that are responsible for coordinating and controlling all of your organs, bodily functions, muscular contractions, as well as allowing you to feel sensations. Your spine is protecting some pretty important stuff.

SPINAL MOVEMENTS

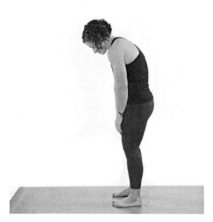

Spinal Flexion.

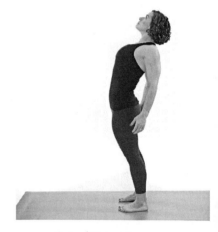

Spinal Extension.

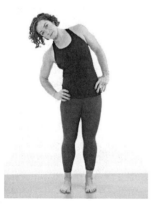

Lateral Spinal Flexion (right).

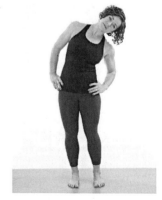

Lateral Spinal Flexion (left).

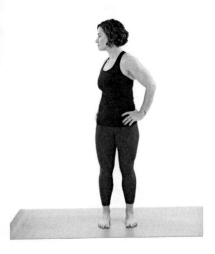

Spinal Rotation (right).

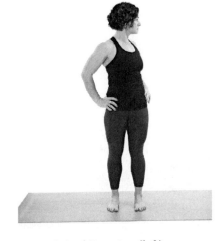

Spinal Rotation (left).

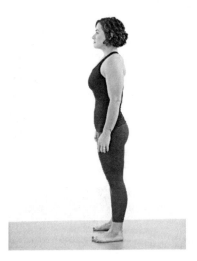

Axial Extension.

A healthy spine can move in seven ways:

- Spinal Flexion: occurs when you round your spine and slump forward
- Spinal Extension: occurs when you arch your back and bend backward
- Lateral Spinal Flexion to the right: occurs when you lean to the right

- Lateral Flexion to the left: occurs when you lean to the left
- Spinal Rotation to the right: occurs when you twist to your right
- Spinal Rotation to the left: occurs when you twist to your left
- Axial Extension: occurs when you lengthen upward as you stand or sit up to your full height

Your spine has to be flexible enough to allow for all these movements while still providing a protective encasement for your spinal cord. This creates an interesting dynamic. In order for your spine to protect your spinal cord, when it moves, it has to move uniformly and as a single cohesive unit. But there's a catch. Each segment of your spine has unique features and shapes that do not allow for completely uniform movement across all segments and, as a result, each segment has different movement potential and structural limitations built into it.

In the thoracic spine, your ribs are attached to all 12 of your thoracic vertebrae, which creates limitations on movement since your ribs come together in front to form your rib cage. Since your rib cage is there to protect the vital organs that live inside it—your heart and lungs—you can see that the instinct in this section of your spine is to favor preservation of life over mobility. Additionally, the bony knobs on the back of the spine, called the spinous processes, in your thoracic spine point downward, which means that there isn't much potential for back bending here before those bones start bumping in to each other. This explains why so many of us feel "locked up" in this area of our spines.

On the other hand, in your lumbar spine, we see a different dynamic. First, none of the lumbar vertebrae are directly connected to your ribs or pelvis. Also, in this segment of the spine, the discs are thicker, and there is significantly more space between the spinous processes. For those reasons, there's a lot more movement potential here and thus a tendency to overrely on it. This is often referred to as "laying in" your lower back—a phrase commonly used to describe hanging out in your end range of motion in lumbar extension where the facet joints are literally leaning into each other, compressing the cartilage, and producing that familiar feeling of achiness. Your bones aren't meant to always be leaning into each other but as you get tired and slouch, your core muscles relax and your spine slips into its end range of motion, relying on the passive structures in your spine to keep you upright and bear the weight of your upper body.

Because of the importance of continuity of movement among the segments of your spine and considering the significant inherent limitations within certain segments, we need a sophisticated system of support that can create constant and precise adjustments to the position of the individual pieces of the spine. Lucky for you, you have a whole bunch of muscles in the space between your ribs and pelvis to help—assuming you learn how to use them skillfully.

The Core Muscles

When most people hear "core," what they really think is "abs," but we're going to paint a much broader picture than that. We'll define "the core" as all the muscles that form the entire circumference of your torso in the space between the bottom of your rib cage and the top rim of your pelvis. So what we're talking about here is:

- Rectus Abdominis: your primary spinal flexor, which runs from the bottom edge of your rib cage near your sternum, down the front of your core, and attaches to your pubic bone
- Internal and External Obliques: your primary spinal rotators, together these two sets of muscles form a big "X" across your abdomen and around the sides of your waist—your external obliques run from the sides of your rib cage to the area near your belly button and your internal obliques run from the side of your pelvis to the area near your belly button
- Quadratus Lumborum: your primary lateral flexors, which attach to the back of your lower ribs, down your lumbar spine, and connect to the bony rim of the back of your pelvis
- Transverse Abdominis: your deepest layer of abdominal support, which forms a thin sheath that runs from one side of your lumbar spine, covering the entire surface of your abdomen from rib cage to pelvis, all the way around to the other side of your spine
- Erector Spinae: your primary spinal extensors, which attach to the base of your skull, continue all the way down your back, and connect into the back of your pelvis
- Diaphragm: your primary breathing muscle, which sits up inside your rib cage and forms the top of your abdominal cavity

- Psoas: these muscles sit beside your lumbar spine forming critical pillars of support to your lower back as well as creating the curve of your lumber spine
- Pelvic Floor Muscles: these muscles offer support to all your abdominal organs and form the bottom of your abdominal cavity

You may think of the core as being the muscles that move your spine. That is certainly true. However, if these muscles were powerful movers of your spine, your spinal cord could be damaged. Instead, their role in creating functional movement is really more about creating cohesion in the way your spine moves—distributing the demand over several joints to create continuity. This intelligent unification and redistribution is what decreases the amount of localized hyperflexion (rounding forward) and hyperextension (overarching) so that there's no pinching or damage to the spinal cord. In other words, the real magic of your core is its ability to resist and contain movement as well as provide the necessary stabilization support to each of its joints in order to keep the bones of your spine from bumping each other, the discs between them, or your spinal nerves.

In your thoracic spine, your ribs provide passive stabilization and typically do a good job of keeping your thoracic vertebrae from moving enough to damage your spinal cord. You don't have to think about it in your thoracic spine because the containment is built into the skeletal structures. In your lumbar spine, that's the job of your core. You have to pay attention and actively participate in the process of stabilizing your lower back. These muscles need to be supportive enough to have the capability to resist movement but also be flexible enough to allow the individual segments of the spine to move in proportion to the rest of the structure. In other words, you need balance. It's a community of muscles that needs to be trained to work well together, which is exactly what you'll learn to do in this chapter.

Let's look at how your core muscles actually accomplish this. Each muscle of your core is capable of creating a specific motion in your spine. For example, your rectus abdominis (the "six-pack" muscle) connects the bottom of your sternum to your pubic bone and is responsible for creating spinal flexion—the vigorous muscular contraction we know as "crunching." This action in and of itself is not particularly functional when you consider that poor posture and gravity are already pulling us that way for large portions of the day. So training this movement is not really all that helpful. However, when you think of these muscles less as prime movers and more as prime stabilizers, you see that their true superpowers don't lie in vigorous, all-or-nothing contractions, but rather in skillful and precise adjustments to the position of your lumbar spine that ultimately bring it into alignment with the rest of the structure. Circling back to the example of the rectus abdominis, its true functional role is in drawing your front ribs down and lifting the front rim of your pelvis up to decrease the amount of compression in the facet joints at the back of your spine. But if this action is taken to the extreme, the discs at the front of the spine become compressed. Again, it's all about balance. You need enough engagement to protect one side of your spine but not so much that you compress the other side.

Obviously your core muscles have some other very important functions, such as:

- creating respiration (breathing);
- protecting, supporting, and drawing the contents of your abdomen in toward the weight-bearing support of your spine; and
- helping to facilitate efficient movement and energy transfer;

but isometric and dynamic stabilization will be our focus, as stabilization is the most important function of your core for creating durability in your spine.

Common Issues Among Runners

When running, the direct role of your core in moving you forward is limited. Instead, your core's primary role is stabilizing your spine—controlling motion where it would be uncomfortable or inefficient—and maintaining an upright running posture. Poor postural habits and gravity can thwart the core in fulfilling its role. Many of us spend large portions of the day sitting or slouching, which creates imbalance among the muscles that support the spine. When the muscles aren't sufficiently supportive, we lean into the more passive joint structures like the discs, cartilage, or the bones themselves, and things start to ache. Then we take this slouched posture and add in the impact of running and create a recipe for disaster.

When you're running, this shows up as a tendency to let the pubic bone and front hip points tilt downward and the front ribs to lift upward. This lengthening of the muscles at the front of your core can lead to compression in your lower back. Then, as you fatigue, your shoulders start to roll forward, causing strain in the erector spinae muscles that run from the base of your skull all the way down to the back of your pelvis.

Additionally, your efficiency as a runner depends heavily on your ability to effectively manage and control the amount of rotation that naturally occurs in you torso as you run. You may not think of running as involving much rotation, but it does. As your right leg swings forward in your running stride, so does your left arm. Then, as your left leg swings forward, your right arm swings forward as well. Every step creates rotational forces in your torso. The joints in your lower back and pelvis are not designed to allow for much twisting or rotation, so these forces need to be managed and absorbed by your core muscles to minimize the cumulative effect on your joints. With every step of your running gait, your core is working to absorb and limit the amount of twisting. When your core is unable to effectively absorb these rotational forces, energy is wasted, your running form suffers, your lower back and hips may start to ache, and running feels a whole lot tougher than it needs to.

KEY POINT:
Practice Core Engagement for Running Without Holding Your Breath

Sometimes my clients don't understand how to engage the core and take full breaths in and out at the same time. I imagine this is another consequence of the commonly-held, yet erroneous, belief that the vigorous crunching action of rectus abdominis is the same thing as "core engagement." Or perhaps it comes from thinking that "engage your core" means "suck it in," or that your belly must move in order for a breath to be full. In those scenarios, yes, it would most certainly be difficult to continue to breathe while trying to maintain the contraction. But that's not what we're talking about when referring to core activation. Remember, the action we're after is far more subtle. It's the product of an entire community of muscles working cooperatively, not one muscle contracting vigorously in isolation.

Let's look at what's involved in the action of breathing and how it relates to your core. Your primary breathing muscle is your diaphragm, which sits up inside your rib cage like a parachute. When you take a breath in, the muscle fibers of your diaphragm shorten and contract to pull your diaphragm down toward your abdomen to create a vacuum that draws air into your nose or mouth and into your lungs. This is your inhale. Then, the muscle fibers relax and allow your diaphragm to soften back up into your ribs to press air out of your lungs. This is your exhale.

If you were to exaggerate and deepen your breath, you'd notice that the shape of your belly distorts on your inhale. This happens as your diaphragm extends lower down toward your abdomen creating a pressurized situation where the shape of your belly extends slightly outward. As you can imagine, this is the opposite effect of the cinching action you get from activating your transverse abdominis.

So how do you take a full breath in while activating the support functions of your deep core muscles? Simple—learn to breathe outward into your lower ribs. Try this exercise.

Seated Strap Breathing

Sit comfortably and wrap a strap (or belt) around the lower part of your rib cage. Cross the ends of the strap in front of you and take up the slack so

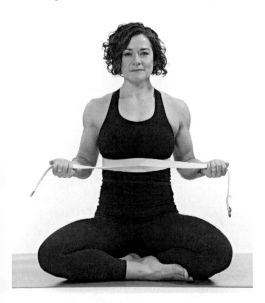

the strap is snug but not tight. Sit up tall and gently engage your transverse abdominis by cinching in around your waist to gently draw the contents of your abdomen toward your spine. Take a full breath in and—rather than directing your breath all the way down in a way distorts the shape of your belly—expand the bottom of your rib cage and think about pressing your lower ribs out into the strap. As you exhale, feel the ribs draw back into the midline of your body. Repeat for a 10–20 full breaths.

Seated Strap Breathing https://youtu.be/QI AnF3CAf7E

How to Fix It

To run strong and pain-free, you have to (1) preserve the ability of your spine to move in all directions; (2) consciously relax the tissues that have a tendency to be tight; (3) manually stimulate the areas that have a tendency to be strained for better circulation to and reoxygenation of the tissues; and (4) train the muscles of your core to work cooperatively to better support the neutral curve of your lumbar spine.

The Movement Practices
Mobilize and Release Your Spine

Since we know that gravity and slouching are already pulling us into rounding forward, it's good to balance all that out with mobility work that maintains range of motion in the other planes of movement such as back bending, side bending, and twisting—which is what we'll do in this section. When it comes to spinal mobility, the point isn't to crank yourself into deeper ranges of motion, it's to be able to move enough to be functional. For that reason, the mobility work prescribed here is pretty passive and gentle. There are built-in structural limitations in your spine, which are there for good reason and should not be disturbed.

Additionally, it's important to note that the lack of mobility that's largely structurally inherent in your thoracic spine (due to the connections to the rib cage) in combination with the relative ease with which you can move your lumbar spine can ultimately cause some overuse issues. What happens then is that you always look to the lumbar spine for movement rather than actively working to maintain the range of motion that your thoracic spine should have. If you don't use it, you lose it, and this places additional demand and strain on your lumbar spine. So we'll also spend some time here working on thoracic spine mobilization as well, which can ultimately do wonders for your running posture.

EQUIPMENT/PROPS NEEDED: Two blocks, a blanket, a bolster, and a foam roller.

Supported Chest Opener
Set up two blocks and a bolster as shown—the block that is furthest from you is at the tallest height and the closer block is at the middle height

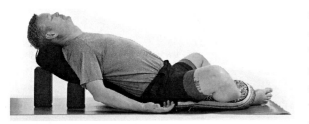

Supported Chest Opener.

and the bolster lays over them both so that it's situated on an incline. Sit facing away from the bolster with your hips right up against the edge of the bolster, knees bent and feet flat on the floor to begin. Roll up your blanket into a long, thin roll. Bring the soles of your feet together and drop your knees out to the sides. Lay the middle of the blanket roll over the tops of your feet and tuck the edges around under your thighs in order to provide support and decrease the intensity of the inner thigh stretch. Then lie back onto the bolster and rest your arms at your sides or in any position that feels comfortable. Stay for 5–10 minutes.

SUPINE TWIST

Lie on your back and draw your knees in toward your chest with your arms out to the sides. Drop your knees over to the left side. If it's difficult to get your knees to the floor or if you feel like the twist is too intense and you can't relax here, put a block under your knees for more support. Another option if

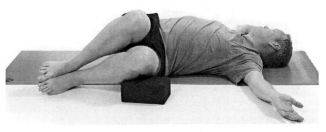

Supine Twist.

this is causing discomfort in your outer right hip, is to put a block or a blanket between your knees. Stay here for 5–10 breaths and then take your knees to the right and repeat.

BANANA

Lie on your back with legs extended long and your arms resting on the floor overhead. Grab onto your right wrist with your left hand and walk your shoulders and head toward the left side of your mat—your shoulders, head, and arms should all be supported by the floor or a prop. Once you're settled there, walk your legs over to the left side of your mat as well and cross one leg over the other (doesn't matter which is on top, try it both ways and do the one you like better). Keep both sides of your hips and shoulders on the floor so that your body

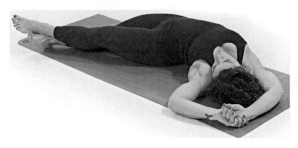

Banana.

is squared to the ceiling above you. Stay here for 5–10 breaths and then bring your legs followed by your shoulders and head back to center and switch sides.

THORACIC SPINE MOBILIZATION

Position a foam roller (or a similarly-shaped blanket roll) across your upper back, about level with your shoulders. Interlace your hands behind your head and rest your head back into them. Keep your hips on the floor and instead of just leaning all the way back (as is the common practice), minimize the arch in your lower back as you let your lower back drop a bit toward the floor and use your abdominals to maintain this position in your lumbar spine by drawing your pubic bone and low ribs slightly toward each other. Keep the engagement of your core here to minimize the tendency for the extension to come from the lumbar spine—imagine not letting your low back lift away from the floor at all as you lean back over the foam roller. You will not go far before your low back lifts into an arched position but if you maintain the support of your core, you'll feel that the small range of motion here comes from your middle back extending over the roller, not from your lower back arching up. Stay for a few breaths then move the roller down to the middle of your shoulder blades and repeat.

Lastly, move the roller down to the bottom edges of your shoulder blades and repeat.

Note: the objective for this work is to mobilize the thoracic spine (mid back), not the lumbar spine (low

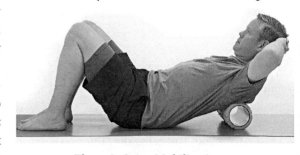

Thoracic Spine Mobilization.

back), so the range of motion is pretty small—more range of motion here is not better. Your hips should remain on the floor and your low ribs should not flare out.

TABLE THORACIC SPINE ROTATIONS

Come into all fours on your hands and knees with your wrists under your shoulders and your knees under your hips. Draw your pubic bone and low ribs slightly toward each other to engage the muscles at the front of your core to support the curve of your lumbar spine. Cinch in around your waist as you stretch to your full height from tailbone to the crown of your head. Place your left hand behind your head and tap the pointy part of your left elbow to your right inner elbow or forearm. Then, take your left elbow back out to

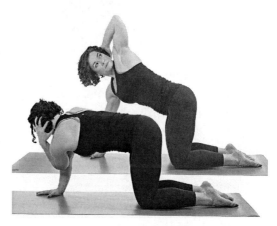

Table Thoracic Spine Rotations.

the left and up toward the ceiling as you broaden through your collarbones. Rotate back to tap your left elbow to your right arm and repeat. Do 8–10 slow rotations per side.

Roll and Release Your Core

It's critical that you're able to maintain the balance between flexibility and stability in this region of the body and to do that you have to create more ease in the muscles that tend to hold onto tension.

In this section, we'll focus on easing existing tension in your muscles by applying some gentle compression in order to manually stimulate circulation to tissues like the erector spinae muscles which have a tendency to get strained from being lengthened and loaded when you slouch. With better circulation comes increased oxygenation, which is critical for the health and resilience of these tissues that are so important to your ability to sit, stand, and run upright.

Additionally, while we already covered the iliopsoas in terms of its role as a primary hip flexor in the preceding chapter, we'll work on it a little bit in this section as well. The iliopsoas is an important pillar of support for your lumbar spine but it has a tendency to get tight. When your iliopsoas muscles get tight, they pull your lumbar spine forward into hyperextension which—as we now know—can compress the facet joints in the lumbar spine. Because of the ability of your iliopsoas muscles to affect the shape of your lumbar spine, it's definitely worth a revisit here.

EQUIPMENT/PROPS NEEDED: Two myofascial balls and a double myofascial ball (optional if you have it).

Erectors

Lie on your back with your knees bent and feet flat on the floor. Place a double myofascial ball or a pair of myofascial balls side by side, one on either side of your spine, just below the bottom of your rib cage. Place your hands behind your head for support. Keep medium pressure on the balls as you gently compress and roll a bit on the tissues. When you find a tender spot, pause there and take a few breaths. Slowly work your way down until you reach the back of your pelvis, pausing

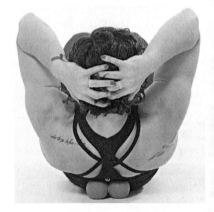

Erectors https://youtu.be/sipcLMvs6z8

to take a few breaths anywhere along the way that feels achy when compressed. After a minute or so, remove the myofascial balls and take a moment to lie on your back and notice the effects of this work.

Quadratus Lumborum

For this work, you'll be covering a similar area as you did above for the erector spinae muscles, except that here the balls will be an inch or two apart on opposite sides of your spine. Lie on your back with your knees bent and feet flat on the floor. Place a pair of myofascial balls side by side with an inch or two between them, one on either side of your spine, just below the bottom of your rib cage. Keep medium pressure on the balls as you gently compress and roll a bit on the tissues. When you find a tender spot, pause there and take a few breaths. Slowly work your way down until you reach the back of your pelvis, pausing to take a few breaths anywhere along the way that feels achy when compressed. Once you get to the back of your pelvis, keep your hips heavy on the myofascial balls and slowly sway your hips from side to side. It should feel like you are dragging the balls over the fibrous tissues there that connect into the back of your pelvis. If you find a tender spot, pause there and take a few breaths as

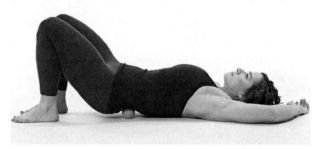

Quadratus Lumborum https://youtu.be/-AUdw_a2Gpc

you gently compress the tissues. After a minute or so, remove the myofascial balls and take a moment to lie on your back.

ILIOPSOAS

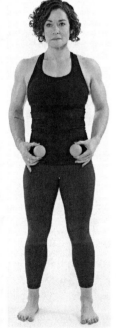

Lie face down on the floor and place the myofascial balls just above and a little to the inside of the bones at the front of your hips (ASIS). Your iliopsoas muscles are deep under your abdominal muscles so the goal is to let your core muscles relax so you can get to your iliopsoas muscles underneath. To do that, spend a few rounds of breath here where you consciously contract the muscles at the front of your core on your inhales and relax them on your exhales. After you've connected to and started to relax your core muscles, you can stop contracting and releasing and instead just focus on continuing to soften your core and let the balls penetrate deeper into the tissues in your pelvis as your body gets heavier. Stay for 10 breaths then remove the myofascial balls and roll onto your back to pause and notice the way your pelvis and lower back feel.

Ball Placement for
Iliopsoas SMR.

Iliopsoas https://youtu.be/oFVFZHMBV4w

Balance and Strengthen Your Core

Most runners I've met have sufficient core strength but what they need is more core control—the ability to better support the natural curve of their lumbar spines while standing, sitting, and running. These muscles in your core are there to subtly position your spine so that things don't bump into other things and cause pain. So, generally speaking, it's ultimately not really an issue of lack of strength but rather a need for more skillful engagement. As a runner, it's imperative that you know how to engage your core muscles to support your spine and have the ability to maintain that support as you move.

Our focus in this section will be on creating the core control necessary to control and—when necessary—adjust the position of your lumbar spine. We'll use isometric holds to build a stronger mind-muscle connection to these muscles and then we'll train them to maintain optimal lumbar positioning as parts of your body move.

IMPORTANT NOTE: functional core work should not be painful. If you are experiencing lower back pain while doing these exercises, or immediately after, it's likely that you are not properly supporting your spine enough in that position. People sometimes choose a more advanced version of the exercise and stick their hands under the back of their hips to keep their low back from hurting. Please stop doing this. Sticking your hands under your hips is a fine short-term solution that decreases the amount of hyperextension in your lumbar spine, but it does nothing to correct the lack of core control that's creating the discomfort there. If your lower back is complaining when you move, it's most likely trying to tell you to engage the front of your core just a little bit more (think bottom ribs and pubic bone gently drawing toward each other). Learn to back off the movement to something you can do without pain, then work on building the skill necessary to progress the movement without causing discomfort in your spine. Work smarter, not harder.

EQUIPMENT/PROPS NEEDED: A long resistance band, a stability ball, and a block.

Stability Ball Dead Bug

Lie on your back with your knees bent and positioned over your hips, shins parallel to the ground. Using your forearms, brace a stability ball against your thighs. Draw your pubic bone and low ribs slightly toward each other to engage the muscles at the front of your core and gently press your lower back into the floor. As you inhale, straighten your left leg out and extend your right arm over your head. As you move, the key is to keep the front of your core engaged

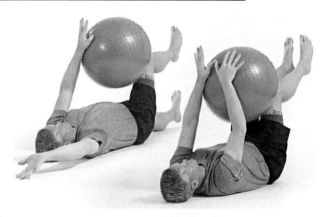

Stability Ball Dead Bug.

and your lower back pressing into the floor. Move slowly enough that you can detect if your lower back arches away from the floor or your lower ribs flare. With your exhale, slowly return your left leg and right arm to the starting position and repeat with your right leg and left arm. It's easy to just go through the motions on this one, so move slowly and really pay attention to whether your core is properly stabilizing your spine. This is about quality of engagement and stability, not range of motion. Perform 3–5 sets of 10 reps per leg, alternating sides.

BLOCK HOLD REACH

Lie on your back with your knees bent and positioned over your hips. Grab a yoga block and place it between your left thigh and left forearm with your left fingers reaching toward the ceiling. Imagine that there was another block on your right side and make the right side of your body match the left side. Draw your pubic bone and low ribs slightly toward each other to engage the muscles at the front of

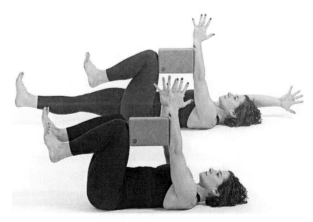

Block Hold Reach.

your core—feel the contact of your lower back to the floor and do not let it change through the movement. Press your left arm and leg into the block as you extend your right arm over your head and reach your right leg away from your head. It's not necessary that your right foot or hand touch the floor—the goal is to keep your spine braced and pressing down into the floor as you move your arm and leg away from each other. Perform 3–5 sets of 10 reps per side.

SIDE PLANK

Lie on your left side with your right foot stacked on top of your left foot and your left elbow under your left shoulder. Keep your feet engaged and your ankles flexed as you lift your hips up away from the floor into a

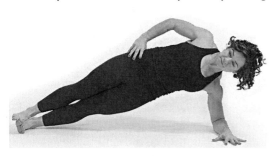

side plank. Actively press the floor away and keep your left side ribs lifting up so that you don't sag into your shoulder. Don't let your hips drift back behind you—remember to engage the front of your core to draw your pubic bone and low ribs slightly toward each other to keep your lower

Side Plank.

back long and not arched. Hold this position for 30 seconds. Then slowly lower down and switch to the other side. Perform 3–5 sets of 30-second holds per side.

Once you've mastered that and can maintain the position easily for 30 seconds at a time, try holding the side plank while "marching"—bring your top knee toward your chest and back without letting your hips sink toward the floor or drift behind you.

HOLLOW BODY HOLD PROGRESSIONS

Lie on your back with your knees bent and positioned over your hips, shins parallel to the ground. Rest your arms on the floor at your sides. Draw your pubic bone and low ribs slightly toward each other to engage the muscles at the front of your core as you press your entire lower back into the floor. Lift your arms and shoulders up just a few inches off the ground, extend your arms over your head, and hold this position for 30 seconds. Keep the front and back of your neck long, in a neutral position, and as relaxed as possible—look up slightly rather than forward to reduce any strain in your neck. Do not let your lower back lift away from the floor. Perform 3–5 sets of 30-second holds.

Once you are easily able to hold this position without letting any part of your lower back lift off the floor, you can increase the challenge by straightening your legs out, squeezing them together, and lowering them to hover a few inches off the floor. If you have any discomfort in your lower back, or if your lower back lifts at all off the floor, bend your knees a bit so that you can keep your lower back pressing down into the floor without discomfort. Remember that the goal here is to create the core strength necessary to keep your lower spine from arching so the moment you feel the arch happening, stop. Work up to 3–5 sets of 30-second holds.

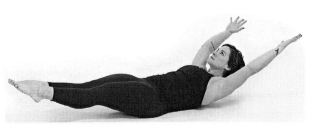

Hollow Body Hold Progressions https://youtu.be/nQT zaE3oSrw

Locust

Lie face down on the floor with your legs extended straight out from your hips with your forehead resting on the floor. Place your arms at your sides with your palms facing down. Without lifting any part of your body off the floor, first lengthen out your body by reaching forward through the top of your head and back through your toes. Draw your pubic bone and low ribs slightly toward each other to engage the muscles at the front of your core—this will help keep you from compressing your lower back. Maintain that engagement at the front of your core and keep actively drawing your ribs back away from the floor as you lift your head, chest, arms, and legs up to hover just off the floor. Rather than trying to lift

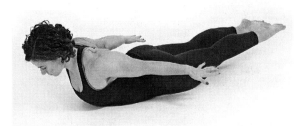

Locust.

your chest and legs high or creating a vigorous clenching contraction of muscles, you're looking for the feeling of global activation where the whole back of your body is working together as a community to lift you. Perform 3–5 sets of 20-second holds.

Antirotational Hold

Anchor one end of a resistance band to something sturdy at chest level. Move far enough away from the anchor point that you feel mild tension on the band when holding the unanchored end of the band with both hands right at the center of your chest. Stand with your feet directly under your hips and draw your pubic bone and low ribs slightly toward each other to engage the muscles at the front of your core. Feel the action of cinching in gently around your ribs as

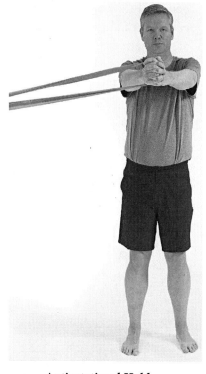

Antirotational Hold.

you stand to your full height. Extend your arms straight out in front of you and hold this position without letting your hands drift away from the midline of your body. Perform 3–5 sets of 30-second holds on each side.

To make this more challenging, step further away from the anchor point. Once you've mastered that, try this hold with a split stance by stepping the leg that's further from the anchor point back into a shallow lunge and then forward again without letting the position of your arms move away from the center line of your body.

Notes on Running Form

The proper upright positioning of your spine and torso helps maximize your lung capacity and plays an important role in the power and length of your running stride. The work laid out in this chapter should help you become more aware of how you position your spine when you're running and give you some great tools to help you find better balance among the muscles that support you. Now let's wrap up this chapter by taking a look at how you can put this all into action in your running form.

- **Do run tall, stretched to your full height.** If you feel yourself start to slouch at any time, take a deep breath in (you'll feel yourself naturally straighten up) and then hold that upright posture as you exhale. Remember that engagement of your erectors to stand up tall and the transverse abdominis to cinch in are things that really just require mindfulness and practice.
- **Do keep your pubic bone slightly lifted.** This will help keep your lower back in a neutral and supported position.
- **Don't let your ribs poke out.** The bottom of your rib cage should rest in a neutral position where the front and back of your core feel equally long and strong.
- **Don't let your shoulders come forward of your ribs.** This will make it much harder to get breath into your lungs.

Key Point:
Lower Back Pain Relief

The work prescribed in this chapter will help you build the capacity and endurance of your core to better control the position of your lumbar spine. In the meantime, if you feel that familiar achy feeling after a run or at the end of your day, it can help to take a few moments with your lower back in a different position to help reset it. Try this out, it's one of my favorites.

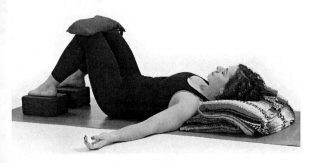

Lower Back Reset.

Lie on your back with your knees bent

and the soles of your feet resting on a pair of yoga blocks. If you have a small sandbag or something similar, place it over your knees for a sweet grounding effect on your legs and hips. Stack two folded blankets as shown—one where the edge is just under your upper back and shoulders and the other on top and just under your head. Set a timer for 5–10 minutes, let your whole lower back lean into the floor, relax, and breathe.

Part 4: Shoulders, Upper Back, and Neck

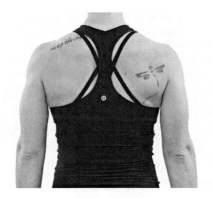

Fix your posture.

For many runners, their shoulders, upper back, and neck are an afterthought. There's so much emphasis in the sport on the lower extremities and core and often little attention is paid to what happens above the waist until things start to go wrong. And when things go wrong up here, they really go wrong—ask anyone who's ever suffered from shoulder and neck pain during or after a run and you'll start to get a clearer picture of just how critical the upper body is to your ability to be happy in running and in life.

Shoulder pain is surprisingly common among runners due to the complexity of the shoulder joint and the repetitive motion of the arms. Even the smallest imbalances, weaknesses, and misalignments around the joint that might not otherwise seem like much of an issue, when coupled with a movement as simple as your arm swing repeated many times throughout your runs, can create significant wear and tear to the joint.

This could result in stiffness in the neck and shoulders, a pinching or dull ache in the shoulder joint itself, or worse—muscle spasms, rotator cuff injuries, or even numbness and tingling down the arm.

But even if you're one of the lucky runners who doesn't have to deal with discomfort during your runs as a result of joint issues or pain in the surrounding tissues here, it's important that you keep reading this chapter anyway. The positioning of your shoulders is also a critical component of running posture and plays a key role in your ability to breathe well. Additionally, your arms and shoulders control, in large part, how much tension is carried in your body. Try this: shrug your shoulders up to your ears and hold them there for a few minutes. How do you feel? Pretty tense, huh? Imagine trying to run that way.

Poor shoulder mechanics and neck positioning are usually caused by poor posture and the pull of gravity that tends to take over when you're fatigued. This combination results in tightness in the muscles that are responsible for rounding your shoulders forward as well as weakness and inactivity in the muscles that draw your shoulder blades together over the back of your rib cage and help to keep you upright. As with every other section of this book (and your body) the secret to correcting issues in these areas of your body is to create better balance between the muscles that support your joints. Think of it as settling an anatomical tug-of-war.

Anatomy and Physiology Basics

The Glenohumeral (Shoulder) Joint

The glenohumeral joint is your main shoulder joint and it's the place where your scapula (shoulder blade), humerus (upper arm bone), and clavicle (collarbone) come together. It is the most mobile joint in your body, which makes it quite a bit more complicated than your other joints. As you'll see here as we unpack this a bit, a lot has to go right to keep this joint balanced and aligned but gravity and our modern lifestyles are not working in our favor.

The shoulder joint is a ball and socket joint—which means that the head of your humerus (the "ball") rests inside a cup-like structure (the "socket"), similar to the hip joint. The main difference in the shoulder vs. the hip is the amount of surface area on the ball that's covered by the socket. In the hip, the head of your femur is pretty well encapsulated by the acetabulum and surrounding joint structures, making it a pretty snug and stable fit. In the shoulder, that's not the case—there's far less encapsulation of the head of your humerus and therefore much greater movement potential.

Another major difference between the hip and shoulder joints is that the hip socket is one solid piece of bone that doesn't change positions as your femur moves. In the shoulder, the socket—called the glenoid fossa—is formed mostly by the outer and upper edges of your shoulder blade which glides around and over the back of your rib cage. This adds another level of complexity. In order for the head of your humerus to be able to move through its full range of motion, your shoulder blade also has to move. Otherwise, you start having bones running into other bones—and potentially the sensitive soft tissues that pass through this area—at the front of your shoulder. With so many moving pieces relying on the proper function and range of motion of other moving pieces, it starts to become clear why the intersection of these three bones is so complicated.

These structural distinctions contribute to the natural tendency of the shoulder to be a more mobile joint than the hip. For most purposes, this natural tendency toward mobility in the shoulders serves us and our lives well. We need our hips to be stable since they support a large part of our body weight as we sit, stand, and move through our lives. Our shoulders, on the other hand, generally aren't used all that much for weight bearing. Since we do so much in our lives with our hands, it's really important that we have mobility in our shoulders that allows for the precision of using our arms—and by extension our hands and fingers—to interact with the world around us.

Shoulder Movements

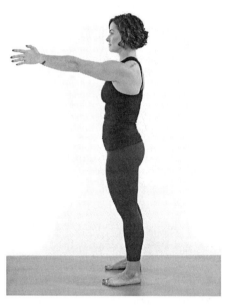

Shoulder Flexion.

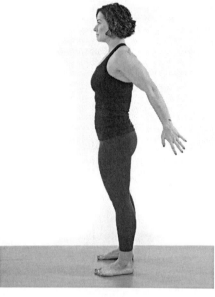

Shoulder Extension.

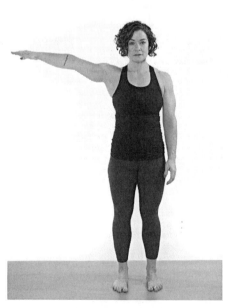

Shoulder Abduction.

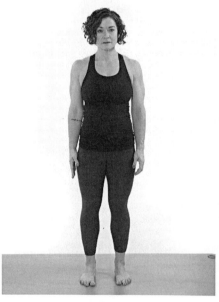

Shoulder Adduction.

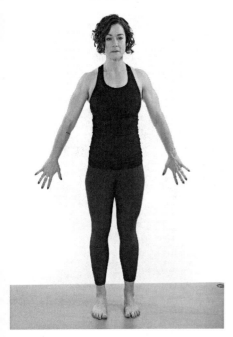 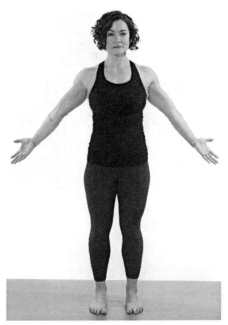

Shoulder Internal Rotation.   **Shoulder External Rotation.**

A healthy, balanced shoulder is capable of allowing the upper arm bone to move in six ways:

- Shoulder Flexion: occurs when you reach your arm forward
- Shoulder Extension: occurs when you reach your arm back behind you
- Shoulder Abduction: occurs when your arm lifts out to the side and away from the midline of your body
- Shoulder Adduction: occurs when your arm moves in toward the midline of your body
- Shoulder Internal Rotation: occurs when your upper arm bone rotates forward in the socket, turning your palm to face behind you
- Shoulder External Rotation: occurs when your upper arm bone rotates back, turning your palm to face forward and slightly upward

Remember that in order to accomplish each of the movements above, a bunch of things have to go right. Specifically, your shoulder blades also

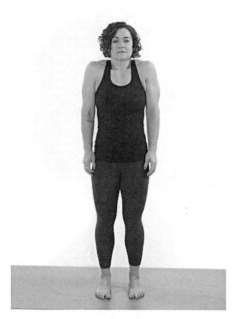

Scapular Elevation.

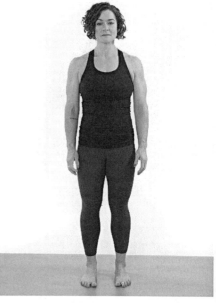

Scapular Depression.

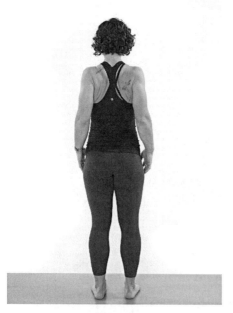

Scapular Retraction.

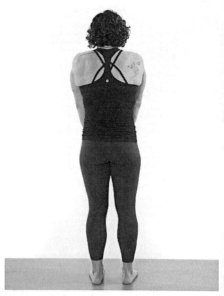

Scapular Protraction.

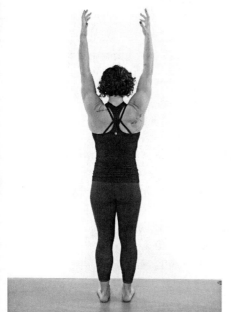

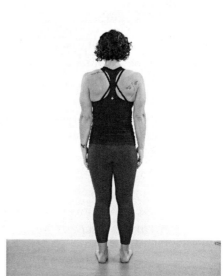

Upward Scapular Rotation.   Downward Scapular Rotation.

have to glide smoothly over the back of your rib cage in a very specific way to accommodate the movement of your upper arm bone. The place where your shoulder blade and rib cage interact is called the scapulothoracic articulation. When things are working well, your shoulder blades can move in one or a combination of six directions:

- Scapular Elevation: occurs when your shoulder blades move upward over the rib cage
- Scapular Depression: occurs when your shoulder blades move downward over the rib cage
- Scapular Retraction: occurs when your shoulder blades move toward each other
- Scapular Protraction: occurs when your shoulder blades move away from each other
- Upward Scapular Rotation: occurs when the bottom tips of your shoulder blades move out away from each other and upward
- Downward Scapular Rotation: occurs when the bottom tips of your shoulder blades move in toward each other and downward

KEY POINT: *Feel It in Action*

Try it out for yourself! See how each movement below changes the positioning of your shoulder blades.

- Scapular Elevation—Stand with your arms naturally hanging by your sides and draw your shoulders up toward your ears.
- Scapular Depression—Pull your shoulders down and away from your ears.
- Scapular Retraction—Squeeze your shoulder blades toward each other on your back.
- Scapular Protraction—Draw your shoulders blades away from each other and round your shoulders forward.
- Upward Scapular Rotation—Take your arms up overhead and the bottom tip of your shoulder blades naturally move outward and upward.
- Downward Scapular Rotation—Bring your arms back down to your sides and the bottom tips of your shoulder blades will naturally move inward and down.

The Shoulder Muscles

In order to maximize the use of all this inherent mobility in your shoulder joint, you come equipped with numerous muscles of varying sizes and capabilities attached to them, similar to puppet strings. For our purposes, we'll classify them into two main groups based on their primary action: the movers and the stabilizers.

First, let's talk about shoulder movers. There are two types of movers: (1) muscles that move your humerus and (2) muscles that move your scapula. These mover muscles of your shoulder are bigger, more superficial, and probably pretty familiar to you: deltoids (front, side, and rear), latissimus dorsi, pectoralis major, biceps, triceps, trapezius (upper, mid, and lower), and levator scapulae.

You also have shoulder stabilizers. These muscles primarily work to position your bones and keep them stable. There are two types of stabilizers: (1) muscles that stabilize the head of your humerus in the socket; and (2) muscles that stabilize your scapula on your rib cage. Because of the more "open-air" joint structure here and the tendency toward mobility in the shoulder, shoulder stability is not guaranteed. Instead of having the bony encapsulation of the joint itself providing the bulk of the stability, like you see in the hip joint, you have to rely on the stabilizer muscles in the shoulder to all be balanced and working together to position the head of the humerus and the shoulder blades well for optimal alignment and function. The stabilizer muscles in the shoulders are smaller, live under the mover muscles, and are probably less familiar to you. In this chapter we'll be looking specifically at the muscles that form the rotator cuff (subscapularis, supraspinatus, infraspinatus, and teres minor), serratus anterior, rhomboids, and pectoralis minor.

As I mentioned earlier, in order for your humerus to move into certain positions such as reaching your arms overhead, your shoulder blade also has to move out of the way to allow for that movement. So coordination of the movers that move both the humerus and the shoulder blade is critical to the health of the joint. This theme of coordination extends also to the stabilizers—the positioning of your shoulder blades affects the positioning of the head of your humerus and vice versa. When these muscle groups aren't balanced and working as a community to both move and stabilize the bones that form your shoulder joint, there is potential for the bones to bump into each other and pinch the soft tissues and nerves that live around the joint.

With so many muscles attaching to and acting on the bones to create movement and stabilize the position of your bones within the joint, many things have to go just right for your shoulder joint to move well. If any one area becomes dominant, or chronically tight, or otherwise does not work well with the surrounding tissues, the positioning and movement of the entire joint becomes compromised and the likelihood of injury increases. Think of it like an orchestra. Every instrument has a role to play, but no single instrument can be overpowering the others and running the show or what was intended to be beautiful music turns into nails on a chalkboard.

Common Issues Among Runners

Most of the imbalance between the muscles and connective tissues around the shoulder joint are products of the posture we spend the majority of our days in. So many of the common tasks we complete during the day are performed with shoulders that are rounded and hunching forward and a slight forward lean in our necks. Chalk it up to all the time spent looking at computers and mobile devices every day.

Over time, this position causes the muscles in the chest, upper back, and neck to get tight. Conversely, the tissues in the middle back and rear shoulder surrounding the shoulder blades become weak and underutilized. From there, it becomes a vicious cycle. Some muscles are so tight they pull on the shoulder bones and other muscles that have antagonist functions are too weak to fight back to maintain optimal shoulder positioning.

Once the joint is misaligned, shoulder movement is compromised. Then, if you take that misaligned shoulder joint and go for a run, the repetitive movement of your arm swing can be enough to create unnecessary wear and tear inside the joint and ultimately cause pain or injury. It's important that you create and maintain balance in and around the shoulder joint so you don't have bones bumping into other sensitive structures.

And even if you're lucky enough to not have it result in a serious shoulder injury, improper alignment of your shoulder is enough to create an inefficient arm swing, make it very difficult to keep your posture upright, and inhibit your ability to breathe fully and properly. This is definitely not a recipe for running well.

KEY POINT: *Set Yourself Up for Running Success by Setting Your Shoulder Blades*

A major key to efficient running posture and having healthy shoulders for life is being able to set your shoulder blades and avoid the dreaded scapular winging—a term that refers to the bottom tips of your shoulder blades lifting up away from your rib cage as their upper edges tilt forward, potentially leading to pinching at the front of your shoulder. Your ability to set and maintain this scapular positioning will also help to create a more efficient arm swing, release unnecessary and unproductive tension in your upper back, and maximize your lung capacity for better breathing. Try this exercise:

1. Gently hug your arm bones down into their sockets.
2. Visualize the inner edges of your shoulder blades gently drawing toward each other and gliding over the back of your rib cage.
3. Broaden through your collarbones but avoid puffing your chest up or letting your lower ribs flare out.

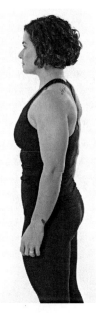

Position your shoulder blades for proper running form and optimal breathing.

Although each muscle within the community is capable of producing some muscular action, it's important to remember that they are designed to work together as a community—skillfully working together to position the bones of the joint and coordinate with each other. To that end, what we're looking for is more subtle or low-grade engagement that can be maintained for longer periods of time as opposed to exaggerated or vigorous contractions of the muscles to create movement.

How to Fix It

To restore optimal alignment to your shoulders, you have to address: (1) the mobility of the tissues that are pulling excessively on your bones, (2) the formation of fibrous adhesions that may have formed between the muscle layers as well as allowing for the recirculation to and reoxygenation of the tighter, more strained tissues, and (3) the conditioning of the weaker, underutilized tissues responsible for holding your bones in their proper position. It's this balance that enables the bones that form the shoulder to align well and glide over and around each other with relative ease and without disturbing the adjacent structures and tissues.

The Movement Practices

Mobilize and Release Your Shoulders,
Upper Back, and Neck

To create greater neutrality here, you have to start by combatting the effects of gravity and poor postural habits. The practice that follows is designed to mobilize, release, and relax the muscles that tend to work overtime and pull you forward into the hunch. Because these muscles tend to be some of the larger and more powerful mover muscles around the shoulder, the goal is to get them to loosen up a bit so that deeper stabilizing muscles can do their part as well. This is how you create efficient movement—by putting every muscle in the community in a position where it can do its job.

It's also worth noting that a lack of mobility in your thoracic spine can contribute to poor alignment in your neck, shoulders, and upper back. You'll find several effective thoracic spine mobilization techniques in the previous chapter.

EQUIPMENT/PROPS NEEDED: Two blocks, a blanket, and a strap.

Supported Blanket Roll Pec Reset

Grab a blanket (or your yoga mat) and roll it up to form a cylinder that's about four inches thick and long enough to support your spine from sacrum to skull. Sit with your knees bent and feet flat on the floor in front of you and place the roll behind you. Sit on the edge of the roll that's closest to your hips and lie back to rest your spine and head on the roll. Place your arms at your sides in a comfortable position where you don't feel much of a stretch at all in the muscles of your chest—you're looking to get the pectoralis major to be relaxed enough that the deeper and smaller fibers of pectoralis minor can release. Extend your legs long or keep your knees bent and feet flat on the floor—perhaps walk your feet a little wider than your hips and let your knees rest in on each other. Close your eyes and visualize your shoulders being able to relax and

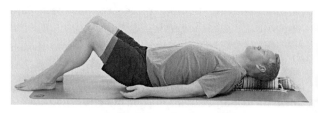

Supported Blanket Roll Pec Reset.

drop down toward the floor with every exhalation. Stay for at least 5 minutes.

PRONE CACTUS STRETCH

Lie face down on your belly and take your right arm out to your right side with your elbow bent to 90 degrees. Take a look over and be

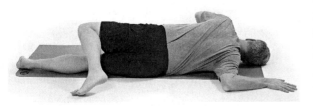

sure that your elbow is level with your shoulder (or perhaps a little higher). Place your left hand under your left shoulder and press down to roll the

Prone Cactus Stretch.

back of your body over toward your right arm until your hips are stacked. Rest your head on the floor or a prop. You can stay there with your legs stacked or bend your left knee and place your left foot on the floor behind you. Stay for 30–45 seconds and then switch sides.

EAR TO SHOULDER ROLLS WITH ELBOW BIND

Sit comfortably with your hands behind your back and grab onto opposite wrists, forearms, or elbows. Drop your chin down toward your chest and relax your shoulders. Slowly start to roll your right ear toward

your right shoulder, pause for a moment, and then roll your head back to center. Then, roll your left ear toward your left shoulder, pause for a moment, and then roll your head back to center. Do a few more rounds of this, alternating sides, pausing anywhere along the way if it feels helpful.

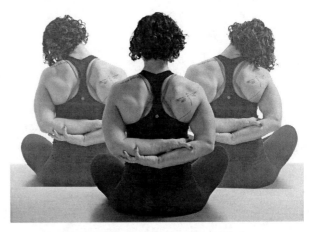

Ear to Shoulder Rolls with Elbow Bind.

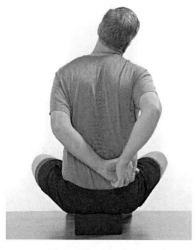

Two-Way Neck Stretch.

Two-Way Neck Stretch

Sit comfortably with your hands behind your back and fingers interlaced. Take both your hands toward the right side of your body and hold them there as you drop your right ear toward your right shoulder. Stay there for 15–20 seconds as you focus on relaxing your neck and shoulders. Then, keep your right ear leaning toward your right shoulder but start to turn your chin down toward your collarbone. Hold there for another 15–20 seconds. Slowly return your head to the starting position and repeat on the other side.

Strap Side Bends

Sit comfortably and hold a strap (or belt) in front of you with your palms facing down and hands more than shoulder-width distance apart. Take your arms up overhead and pull on the strap with your hands a little bit as you lean over toward your right. Stay for a few rounds of breath and repeat by leaning to your left side.

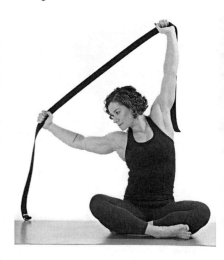

Strap Side Bends.

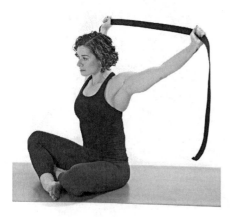

Strap Pull.

Strap Pull

Sit comfortably and hold a strap (or belt) over your head, hands just inside shoulder-width distance apart, palms facing forward. Pull the ends of the strap apart with your hands and slowly start to take your arms back until you encounter the first bit of resistance in the form of a stretch through your chest. Hold there for a few rounds of breath and continue to pull on the ends of the strap.

BLOCK SHOULDER STRETCH

Come to your hands and knees and place two blocks on the floor in front of you on the lowest height. The blocks should be about as wide apart as your shoulders with enough space between the blocks to fit your head. Place your elbows on the blocks with the palms of your hands touching and walk your knees back to lower your head and chest toward the floor. Bend your elbows to bring your hands toward the back of your head or neck. If this is too intense, you can: (1) widen the blocks out a bit, (2) reduce the amount of bend in your elbows, or (3) put a prop under

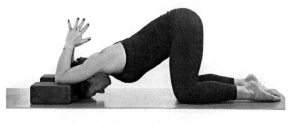

Block Shoulder Stretch.

your head or chest for more support. If this is easy for you, you can increase the height of the blocks. Pick a position where you can stay for 30–60 seconds.

Roll and Release Your Shoulders, Upper Back, and Neck

There are several muscles in and around your shoulders and neck that are known to hold tension. Not only is that tension annoying and often uncomfortable, over time it can lead to movement constriction and improper circulation. In this section, we'll use some gentle compression to these muscles that have a tendency to be tight and overactive. You'll notice that most of the muscles you're working on here are larger and more superficial "mover" muscles; hopefully, if you can get those muscles to relax and soften, it'll ultimately be easier to connect with the smaller "stabilizer" muscles in the strengthening work later in this chapter.

As mentioned earlier in this chapter, there are some sensitive structures running through this area. As you work through these myofascial release techniques, steer clear of anything that feels painful, sharp, or radiates out into other areas of your body. Remember that you're looking for a sensation that is dull and achy but something that you can still relax and soften into.

EQUIPMENT/PROPS NEEDED: Two myofascial balls and a block.

Serratus Anterior, Lats, and Pecs

Lie on your right side and place a block on its middle height with the edge that's closest to you in the right side of your rib cage and the edge that's further from you in your right armpit. Rest your head in your hand. It will feel a little pokey there on your side since there isn't much tissue between the block and your ribs but see if you can relax and soften a bit into it. Stay there for 30 seconds with your shoulders and hips stacked.

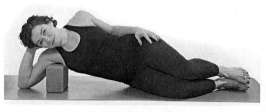

Serratus Anterior SMR https://youtu.be/otwyGq2uruY

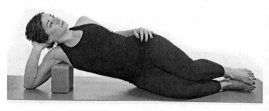

Lats SMR https://youtu.be/otwyGq2uruY

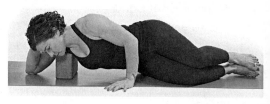

Pecs SMR https://youtu.be/otwyGq2uruY

Then, slowly start to lean your left shoulder back as if you could lean back into the wall behind you. As you do this, the pressure will shift off the muscle tissue at the side of your rib cage (serratus anterior) and onto your lats, the fleshy mound of tissue right behind your armpit. Stay for 30 seconds.

And finally, slowly start to angle your chest toward the floor, shifting the pressure into your pecs. Stay for 30 seconds then roll onto your back and take a moment to notice the effects of this work and the difference in sensation between the two sides of your body.

Upper Traps

Lie on your back with your knees bent and feet flat on the floor. Wedge a myofascial ball under each side of your upper traps near the corner of your neck. Rest your head on the floor. Lift your hips up and place a block under the back of your hips (not in your lower spine) on the lowest or middle height—whichever feels more comfortable for you. You can wiggle your shoulders around a little to find a tender spot where you'd like to stay. For this one, it can be helpful to move your arms around and overhead to find a position where

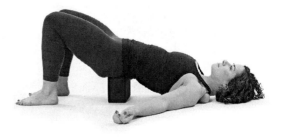

Upper Traps https://youtu.be/siBDYM9u7xE

you feel tenderness in the tissues but let your arms rest on something. Stay in one spot for 30–60 seconds. To come out, remove the balls first, then the block. Lie flat on your back for a moment and observe the effects of this work.

Levator Scapulae

Lie on your back with your knees bent and feet flat on the floor. Position the myofascial balls on either side of your spine near the top inner corner on your shoulder blades—it helps to feel for this spot on yourself while sitting upright first and you'll notice that in this spot, the tissue feels a little bit ropey compared to the textures of the surrounding tissues. Wiggle around a bit and find a spot that feels tender

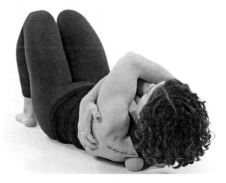

Levator Scapulae https://youtu.be/ PB_aXrQ--lg

and achy and stay for a few breaths. Then, cross your arms over your chest and give yourself a big hug. Rock a little bit from side to side and find a position where you can stay for 30 seconds. Remove the myofascial balls and take a moment to lie on your back. If this feels too intense or if it's challenging to get the myofascial balls in position while lying on the floor, you can do this at the wall instead.

Neck

Lie on your back and place a block at its middle height under your head so that the edge that's closest to your shoulders rests right on the edge of the bony ridge at the back of your skull. Let your arms rest in a comfortable position at your sides. Stay here for about 5–10 breaths and focus on letting your shoulders drop back toward the floor. Then, without lifting your head or shoulders, slowly turn your head all the way to your right. Along the way you'll roll over some thick, rope-like muscles right beside your neck bones. Slowly, keeping your head as heavy as possible on the block, roll about halfway back and

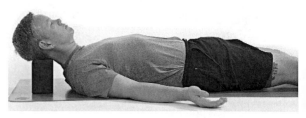

Neck https://youtu.be/T0KhW759kR8

pause anywhere along the way where you feel tenderness. Relax as much as possible to let the block sink in to the tissues. Stay as long as you like on the right side then roll your head back to the center and repeat on the left side. After you've spent a little time with your head turned to the right and left, remove the block and lie on your back for a few breaths.

Balance and Strengthen Your Shoulders

Now that you've introduced a little more mobility to some of the tighter tissues around your shoulders, let's start to create more strength in the muscles that support optimal humeral and scapular alignment within the joint. These muscles are often forgotten about because they tend to serve more stabilizing functions rather than being big mover muscles but they are absolutely necessary for proper shoulder function as well as your ability to maintain an efficient upright running posture.

The corrective work that follows is designed to condition these smaller muscles so that they are active and strong enough to hold the bones of your shoulder in position to allow for a full, healthy range of motion. When everything is balanced and working cooperatively around your shoulders, tension and discomfort start to subside.

EQUIPMENT/PROPS NEEDED: A long resistance band and a dowel.

PRONE ARM PULLS

Lie face down on the floor. Hold a dowel or piece of PVC in your hands with a shoulder-width (or slightly wider) grip, arms extended over your head. Rest your forehead on the floor and lengthen the back of your neck. Press the tops of your feet and thighs into the floor and press your pubic

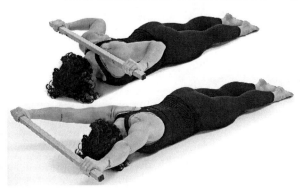

Prone Arm Pulls.

bone down into the floor to engage your low belly (imagine trying to zip up a pair of tight jeans)—this will limit the chances of causing compression in your lumbar spine. Then, keep your head down and low belly engaged and lift your arms and the dowel up off the floor. Bend your elbows and pull the dowel behind your head as close to your shoulders as you comfortably can. Pause for a moment and then straighten your arms to hover off the floor and repeat. Perform 3–5 sets of 10 reps.

SCAPULAR PUSHUPS IN TABLE

Come into all fours on your hands and knees with your wrists under your shoulders and your knees under your hips. Draw your pubic bone and low ribs slightly toward each other to engage the muscles at the front of your core to support the curve of your lumbar spine. Think about creating a subtle cinching in around your waist as you stretch to your full height from tailbone to the crown of your head. Without bending your elbows, draw your shoulder blades together on your back—imagine pinching a pencil between your shoulder blades. Then, do the reverse, draw your shoulder blades away from each other and feel the tissues between your shoulder blades

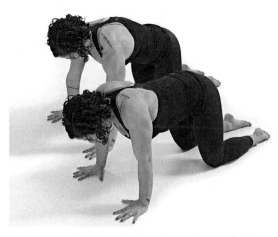

Scapular Pushups in Table https://youtu.be/CCUo-IHpLW4

stretch. The range of motion is small and should be isolated primarily to your upper back. Keep your core engaged and lifted throughout. Perform 3–5 sets of 10 reps.

STRAIGHT ARM PULL DOWN

Anchor a long resistance band to something low, a few inches off the ground will work. Lie on your back with your knees bent, feet flat on the floor. Slide a sturdy dowel or piece of PVC pipe through the resistance band and hold onto it in an overhead position with your hands shoulder-width distance apart. Move far enough away from the anchor point that you feel mild tension on the band. Draw your pubic bone and low ribs slightly toward each other to engage the muscles at the front of your core—use this activation to brace your lower spine through the entire movement. Keep your elbows straight (but not locked out) and your neck long as you press the dowel forward and down toward your hips. Pause for a moment and slowly return to the overhead position with control and without releasing the tension in your lats and core. Perform 3–5 sets of 10 reps. To make this more challenging, move your body further from the anchor point.

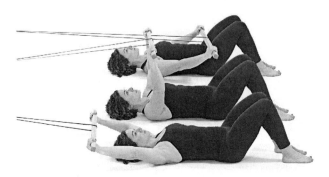

Straight Arm Pull Down.

LAT PULLS

Anchor a long resistance band to something low, a few inches off the ground will work. Lie on your back with your knees bent, feet flat on the floor. Slide a sturdy dowel or piece of PVC pipe through the resistance band and hold onto it in an over-

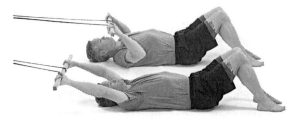

Lat Pulls.

head position with your hands shoulder-width distance apart. Move far enough away from the anchor point that you feel some tension on the band. Draw your pubic bone and low ribs slightly toward each other to engage the muscles at the front of your core—use this activation to brace your lower spine through the entire movement. Bend your elbows and pull the dowel toward the top of your chest. Pause for a moment and then slowly and with control return to the stating position to repeat. Perform 3–5 sets of 10 reps.

If you have access to a pull-up bar or lat pull down machine, those work well for this too.

RESISTANCE BAND PULL APARTS

Stand tall with your feet hip-width distance apart. Grab a long resistance band with your palms facing up, hands should be shoulder-width distance apart and level with the lower part of your chest. Keep your neck long and as relaxed as possible—so that you maintain the space between your shoulders and ears. Pull your hands against the resistance of the band as far away from each other as you can by drawing your shoulders blades together on your back. Pause for a moment then slowly return your hands to the starting position with control to repeat. Perform 3–5 sets of 10 reps.

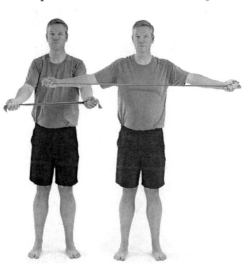

Resistance Band Pull Aparts.

FACE PULLS

Anchor a long resistance band to something stable at shoulder or head height. Grab the band with your palms facing down and leave 4–6 inches

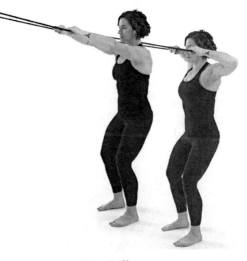

Face Pulls.

between your hands. Step back from the anchor point so that you feel some tension on the band with your arms straight. Position your ankles under your hips and bend your knees slightly into an athletic stance (like you're about to jump). Pull the band back toward your face, keeping your elbows above the height of your shoulders as you draw your elbows back. Pause for a moment then slowly and with control return to the starting position. Don't scrunch up your neck, flare your front ribs, or arch your lower back. Perform 3–5 sets of 10–15 reps.

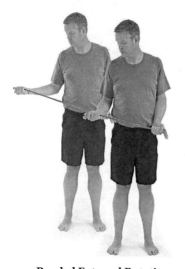

Banded External Rotation.

Banded External Rotation

Hold a resistance band in your left hand right in front of your left hip. Grab the opposite end of the band with your right hand, palm facing up with your elbow bent to 90 degrees and close to your right side. Keep your neck long, right elbow close, and shoulders relaxed as you rotate from your right shoulder to draw your right hand out to your right side against the resistance of the band. Pause for a moment there before slowly and with control returning your hand to the starting position to repeat. Perform 3–5 sets of 10 reps per arm.

Bent Over Band Row

Stand on one end of a long resistance band with your right foot and step your left foot back into a split-leg stance. Grab onto the opposite end of the resistance band with your right hand. Hinge slightly forward from your hips, engage your abdominals by gently drawing your pubic bone and low ribs slightly toward each other. Align your head with your spine in a neutral position. Gently hug your right upper arm

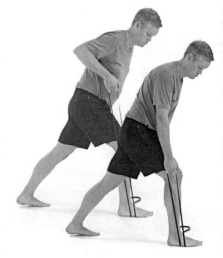

Bent Over Band Row.

bone down and into its socket and maintain this "packed" position through the entire movement. Pull upward on the band as you draw your elbow up and back. Pause for a moment there and slowly return to the starting position without releasing the engagement of the muscles. Perform 3–5 sets of 10 reps per side.

Notes on Running Form

We all need to do a better job when it comes to posture and being mindful of how we spend the majority of our time. The work described in this chapter will get you on the right track for that. But one of the best places for runners to practice better posture is while running—with a particularly strong emphasis during hard effort runs and at the tail end of each run. The better you get at conditioning your muscles to maintain a strong, upright posture when fatigued, the easier and more automatic it will become in daily life.

Keep in mind that the posture you maintain during your runs is form practice—and we always need to be consciously practicing good form and not just relying on our bodies to do it well. So be mindful of the times that you let your form fade as you get fatigued and train yourself to do better. This way, you'll be reinforcing a posture that could ultimately benefit your running times and improve the health of your neck and shoulders.

When you're running, focus on the following key areas to create a better and more efficient running posture. You'll not only feel stronger, but you'll breathe better and be far less likely to find yourself sidelined by shoulder and neck pain and/or injuries.

- **Do run tall, stretched to your full height.** Think about stretching the top of your head up to keep the muscles in your neck active and engaged.
- **Do keep your chin level.** This helps keep the muscles of your neck and upper back relaxed and in a neutral position.
- **Don't let your chin jut out in front of you.** This also helps facilitate a more relaxed position in your neck and upper back.
- **Do look straight ahead.** Your posture usually follows your gaze. Looking down often results in the upper body rounding forward.

- **Do keep your shoulders low and loose.** Create some relaxed space between your ears and shoulders by gently engaging the muscles of your mid-back to gently draw your shoulder blades back and down. This will help you avoid the "high and tight" shoulder positioning.
- **Do keep the tops of your shoulders level.** You want your shoulders to be relaxed but also steady. When your postural muscles are inactive or fatigued, the wrong muscles start taking over and you'll notice a dipping action in your shoulders from side to side with each stride.
- **Do move your arms forward and back.** Avoid letting your arms swing side to side or across your midline. Imagine wearing a zip-up jacket and not letting your hands cross the zipper to the other side of your body.
- **Don't clench your fists.** Your fingers should lightly touch the palms of your hands in unclenched fists as if you were holding a potato chip in your hand that you didn't want to crush. Otherwise, tension in your hands will travel up into your arms, neck, and shoulders.
- **Do breathe into your lower ribs.** Practice using your diaphragm to help you breathe by expanding your lower ribs laterally (out to the sides) rather than breathing shallow and high into your upper ribs and chest. It's important that you learn to access and use this powerful breathing muscle to its full potential. When you don't, the accessory (less efficient) breathing muscles of your neck, chest, and upper back kick in—leading to or perhaps further contributing to tension and tightness in these areas.

KEY POINT:
Practice Relaxed Breathing

When you feel stressed or anxious, the accessory breathing muscles around your neck and shoulders have a tendency to get tense and become overactive. This usually leads to the feeling of increased tension and anxiety. One of the ways you can interrupt this cycle is to reset your breath-

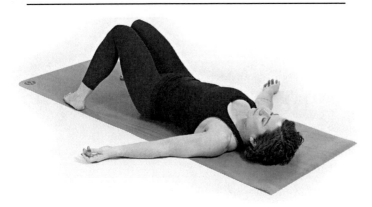

Diaphragmatic breathing allows your accessory breathing muscles around your neck, ribs, and shoulder to relax. https://youtu.be/XxZlJn3LSH0

ing patterns by breathing in a relaxed way from your diaphragm. Try this exercise to relax those smaller muscles around your neck and shoulders.

1. Lie on your back with your knees bent and your feet flat on the floor. Separate your feet so they are slightly wider than your hips and let your knees fall in and rest on each other.

2. Rest your hands comfortably either on your belly or on the floor and grab a blanket if you'd prefer something under your head. You're looking for a position that requires no effort and is easy to drop into so that you can let your body lean into the floor and be really passive.

3. First, just start to observe your breath. Notice where you feel it most—in your chest, ribs, or belly.

4. Then, see if you can direct more of your breath toward your lower ribs and belly. You can even place your hands at your side ribs or belly if you'd like the feedback of feeling your ribs and belly rise and fall.

5. As you inhale, direct your breath down into your lower ribs and belly.

6. As you exhale, let your ribs and skull get a little heavier as all the muscles around them relax.

7. Stay here and breathe for a few minutes to give your shoulders and neck a chance to unwind and soften.

Part 5: Mental Durability

Runners are a committed crew. We spend our time working on our conditioning and endurance, analyzing splits, logging miles, timing out nutrition, and building the strength to carry ourselves where we need to go. We get why the physical stuff matters, and we are willing to put in the work and fight for performance gains. This belief that the hard stuff will make us better keeps us coming back for more and more challenge.

We pour ourselves into physical training because it typically provides the most perceptible corporeal results. We can see and feel the fruits of our efforts in the form of faster times, higher mileage, increased power, reduced rates of injury, and improvements in efficiency. These results are the evidence that makes the process easier to buy into. Everyone likes validation for their efforts, and nowhere is that more obvious than in the way we train our bodies for this sport. We continue to do the things that we know work for us based on the evidence we see.

We also know that physical abilities are trainable. We understand that in order to improve our strength, conditioning, and endurance, we have to train them. The entire field of exercise physiology is dedicated to providing the framework that we use as our roadmap to improvement and increased capacity.

But many of us still leave the mental aspects of training to chance. I've never had to convince a single client that the right physical training could make them better and more durable. However, it's always an uphill battle to convince people that they can increase their mental durability by training it. Most runners forget about mental training, and it becomes the wild card— the thing that always seems to fail in the final moments of the race.

Many runners believe that mental durability is something you're either born with or not. Some even habitually let their belief that they lack mental toughness become the reason for easing up and not pushing through the tough stuff in training. While at times backing off is the right call, it can also be a golden opportunity to practice mental toughness.

That's not to say that everything that happens in your training is something you need to tough out. You simply need to be more discerning about when you tell yourself to suck it up versus letting your system wind down, recover, and catch up. As with all things related to durability, the key is balance. Balance is a constantly moving target. Only you can make the decision about what's best for you in every moment, so it's important that you learn to read your own gauge. That's what you'll learn to do in this chapter—to develop the specific skills and mental dexterity it takes to move fluidly from moment to moment.

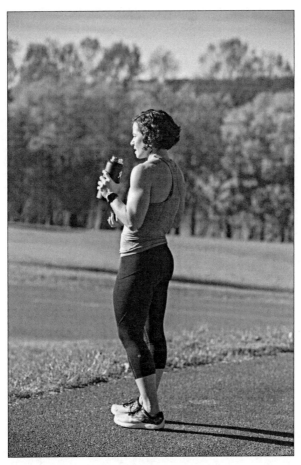

Sometimes you need to push through and sometimes you need to back off. It's up to you to learn to know the difference.

Training for Mental Durability

In the words of the great Amby Burfoot, 1968 Boston Marathon winner and former *Runner's World* editor-in-chief, "If you train your mind for running, everything else will be easy." Runners often fail to train this aspect of durability. It takes a great deal of self-awareness and mental toughness to endure training and competing; without it you burn out, lose motivation, and respond poorly to disappointment.

Your physical training program must be individualized and designed to create adaptation through progressive and specific overloading, with consistent reinforcement, followed by periods of recovery. The same principles apply to mental training. You need an approach that considers your own strengths and weaknesses and is designed to stretch your capacity gradually in a way that is specific to running with time after to mentally decompress as well as repetition to reinforce the skill.

In this chapter, we'll unpack the five key components of mental durability—presence, focus, grit, adaptability, and growth-mindedness—as well as how to train them. At its core, mental durability training is about intentional and deliberate practice. I once heard someone say that during the clutch moments of your life "you cannot summon what you don't possess" and it stuck with me. You have to practice and develop the specific skills you want to have. If you feel like you lack mental durability in the moments when it matters, ask yourself whether you are training in a way that allows you to gain and develop better mental skills or just hoping they'll just show up when you need them.

I find that many runners are just crossing their fingers. Many believe that once they increase their physical abilities, their mental capacity will follow. If that's you, I'm going to save you a lot of time here—you cannot train physically to overcome a poor mindset. Read that again. No amount of mileage will be enough to outrun insufficient mental durability. You have to train both. But I promise you this—if you do, magic will happen.

Cultivating Presence

If you want to do anything in your life well, you have to be present—completely in the moment. Life happens in the now. All the information you need to make good choices is available to you right now. And yet so many of us dwell in regrets from the past or live in fear of the future. Allowing yourself to be constantly split among the past, present, and future is overwhelming—it's far more information than your brain can process or reconcile. The trick is to be where your breath is, because the moment when you realize that the only experience in life you have to manage is the one that's happening now, everything seems more manageable.

Presence is the ability to be in the present moment and take in only the information available to you now, all of it, without being overwhelmed or overly influenced by it. It's the ability to be completely aware of your thoughts and feelings, sensations in your body, and your current environment. When you're able to connect to the present moment and tap into the deepest parts of your human experience, you find the wisdom that already exists inside of you. Some people call it "being in the zone," "flow," or "flow state"—you suddenly know exactly what to do and how to do it, as if your deepest instincts are taking over.

You are a living, breathing, dynamic being. You are constantly changing and adapting. You don't show up as the same you every day with the same capacity for output. How you show up for your runs each day is based on a cocktail of factors like how much sleep you've gotten, your stress and hydration levels, the weather, your emotional state, and your nutritional intake. It's unrealistic to expect that your capacity will be the same day to day. Every day the combination of factors that make you up and influence you are different. Every day you are different.

Presence is intense awareness of your self and the factors that are affecting you in this moment. It sounds so simple, but it can be challenging and uncomfortable to be still and silent long enough to build this awareness. At first, it can be frustrating, as is acquiring any new skill. But this is the first step toward being able to read your own gauge. Practicing presence helps you establish a baseline so you can monitor changes from day to day and detect when something is off. With practice, you start to hone your ability to know the difference between the times to push through and practice toughness and the times to back off and rest. It requires extreme presence. This is where yoga is a powerful tool.

Yoga, mindfulness, and meditation train this skill better than anything else. These modalities offer the tools to help you train yourself to get quiet and still enough that you can see clearly what's right in front of you and step beyond the chatter in your head, your doubts, your regrets, your fears, and your patterns of avoiding struggle. They offer tools to help you develop a new level of self-awareness, so you can make better decisions based on what's happening now rather than past patterns or future predictions. You don't need to be able to right the wrongs of your past, and you don't need to be able to see the future. All that's required of you is to see the information that's currently in front of you and, with that realization, the gravity of what you're facing begins to lessen.

As with most things, in order to develop presence, when you first start out you should practice when it's easy and you're relatively calm so you know what to do when you're being challenged. First thing in the morning is a great time to spend a few moments sitting in meditation to develop your ability to be present. It doesn't have to be fancy or complicated; just five minutes a day can be really powerful. My meditation practice involves setting a timer on my phone, lying on the floor, and settling into the sensation of breath in my body as I imagine that my bones are getting heavier. There's no right or wrong way to meditate, so find ways that work for you. The goal is to simply learn to be where your feet and breath are. Then when you're running and fear of the final miles is overwhelming you, you can find your way back to the present moment by asking yourself "how am I breathing?" or "how is my form?" rather than fighting with future moments of discomfort and struggle that might never come to pass.

KEY POINT:
Learning to Meditate

I usually get initial resistance from my athletes when I tell them to start a regular meditation practice. First, they tell me they don't have time. To that, I say, if you don't have five minutes a day to sit and breathe, then it's time for you to re-evaluate your life choices. Then, as I dig deeper, they tell me that they can't meditate because they cannot turn their brains off. To this, I say thinking is not the enemy.

There is a misconception that you're not meditating unless your head is completely clear. Let that idea go. You're human, and it's your mind's job to think. The point of meditation is to recognize that you are not your thoughts and therefore, you don't have to act on every thought you have. Think of your mind as a clear blue sky and your thoughts as puffy clouds that move across the sky. When you meditate, you simply watch them pop in and out until it becomes clear that your thoughts are just passing through. They are temporary. They don't have to distract you and lead you down the rabbit-hole of thought. They don't have to mean anything other than it's the nature of your mind to generate thoughts.

But thoughts are not the problem. What you do with them and how you let them control you is. There's so much power in being aware of your own inner monologue. Once you're aware of it and you learn to separate who you are from what you're thinking, you discover that you're not stuck with the factory programming. You learn to identify nonproductive thoughts—the thoughts that simply wander aimlessly about in a disorganized way and interfere with your training and your life—and instead choose more productive thoughts.

"Do I have to meditate? Can't I just do this while I'm training?" Well, maybe. It's much easier to see how your mind works while sitting quietly and still. If you can't do it in a still and silent environment, I'm not sure you can do it in the chaos and noise. Remember, "you can't summon what you don't possess." Practice now so you have the skill when the pressure is on.

Refine Your Focus

Goals matter. Without them, there's no purpose to the things you do, and without purpose, there's no fulfillment in life. Your goals are reminders of what's most important to you. At decision points, goals guide you to make better choices, ones that align with something that matters to you.

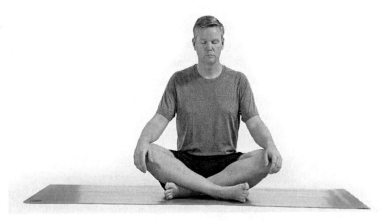

If you can't focus your mind when you're still, it's difficult to do when in motion.

But here's the thing: goals aren't enough. You need actionable items and steps that help you move the dial every day.

Focus is your ability to fix your mind on one thing and tune out the rest. In order to truly focus, the thing you're focusing on has to be specific. Big goals are great, but they aren't going to offer you the exact framework to get you from point A to point B. For that, you need to focus on a specific action.

You certainly need to spend hours practicing your craft to get good at it, but time spent practicing isn't the only factor. It's not enough that you just show up and go through the motions. It's not the number of practice hours that matters most, but the quality of those practice hours. Improvement requires a lot of focused, intentional, and deliberate practice.

I see a lot of runners with big goals get lost in the day-to-day stuff. They have a vision of what they want but forget to pave the road that would lead them there. They show up and log the miles, but it's pretty mindless and unfocused. They're not actually paying attention to and addressing what's really holding them back. There's no intention behind the way they train daily. Having a plan to reach your goals will make you more mentally durable.

At the beginning of every workout, identify something you struggle with and set an intention to practice that thing. For example, if you struggle with fading during the final miles of races, during each of your longer training runs, set the intention to finish strong and practice putting more into the final miles. Don't let yourself slow down and slog through it. Work on keeping your energy and pace up. Stay focused and sharp. Treat the final mile like it's the most important mile you run all week—because it is. In that mile, you have the opportunity to learn to focus through exhaustion, pull your running form together through fatigue, and keep moving forward with strength and intention. This is important because sometimes mile markers are wrong or missing and sometimes your GPS watch will be off. You can choose to spend the final mile of your weekly long run as a chance to practice fading or as a chance to practice finishing. You decide.

If you struggle with negative self-talk, set the intention to practice identifying negative thoughts during your training run and replacing them with something more productive such as a reminder to breathe and run tall. Practice choosing your thoughts the way you choose your target races.

I find it's helpful to take your intention and distill it down to a simple mantra that you can repeat to yourself during key moments. When I ran the NYC Marathon in 2016, it was only seven days after finishing the Marine Corps Marathon—what can I say, it was a lucky race lottery year for me. Of course, I wanted to finish NYC with a decent time—good enough to have my name printed in the *New York Times* the next day at least—but a lot can happen in 26.2 miles, especially when you're running two marathons this close together. So as I stood at the foot of the Verrazzano-Narrows Bridge waiting to be released with my wave onto the course, I closed my eyes and said to myself, "no matter what happens next, be strong." That simple intention—"be strong" provided me with a guide at every decision point along the route—any time I questioned whether I should ease up, I came back to my intention: "be strong." Having that mantra also provided me with a measurement of success that was solidly in my control for the entire race. I did not control the crowds, the weather, the congestion at water stops, or the direction the wind blew—but in every moment of that race, I could choose to be strong and I did. I now encourage all my runners to set a similar intention for all their peak races.

Every workout or training session is an

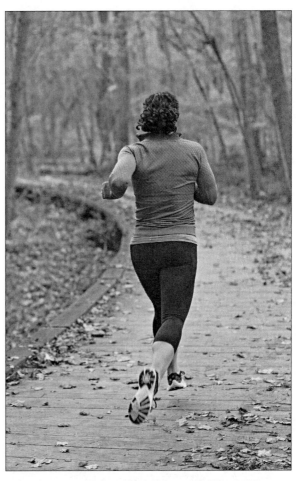

Training is tough, but if you let it, it will make you tougher.

opportunity to practice the skills necessary to move you closer to where you want to be. Don't just go through the motions. Think back to a time when you didn't do as well as you wanted and practice doing better. Create a specific intention to work on and practice holding that focus through the entire workout.

Train for Grit

Into every runner's world, bad runs and races will come. Yet some runners go to extraordinary lengths to avoid uncomfortable training runs—by postponing until the weather clears, cutting the run short when it feels harder than it should, avoiding the route that involves that one big hill, or never programming runs that push them to their edge. If you view every training run that doesn't go according to plan as a sign you should call it a day, you're missing out on many opportunities to refine your grit.

Grit is mental toughness. It's the resolve to push through discomfort and see it through even when things aren't going as planned. In order to develop this skill, you have to train yourself to tolerate and to focus through progressively more challenge and discomfort. It's not a pleasant process, but it is a necessary one. As a coach, it's my job to create programs that intentionally push runners to their limits during training. Part of that is to provoke the physical adaptations necessary to make my runners faster, stronger, and able to go the distance. But the other reason is to make the runner uncomfortable enough that he or she has to develop skills for dealing with discomfort and challenges on the run.

That's the thing about training: it's supposed to train you to be prepared for just about anything. I want things to go wrong during training for my runners. I want them to have to dig deeper mentally in practice—otherwise, how are they supposed to find the will to carry on when it really counts? It's easy to show up and hit your numbers when things are going your way and you feel in control. But it won't make you better.

Some runners coach themselves through their entire marathon training cycle avoiding the type of challenge that might make them uncomfortable and cutting their bad runs short only to fall apart on race day. To be a mentally durable runner, build your grit instead. Don't avoid the tough stuff during your training. Use those times as opportunities to develop the skills for dealing with disaster so that on race day you have tools to keep yourself calm and on track no matter what the day throws at you.

There will always be things you don't control, so practice calling them out on your runs. For example, the next time you have bad (but not dangerous) weather during the time you've set aside for your training run, go anyway. You don't control the weather, but you do control your effort. This way you're prepared for that time when the weather is awful at the start of your race—which will most definitely happen to you someday. Imagine how much more confident you will feel not to obsess over the race day forecast all week because you know you're ready and prepared for whatever Mother Nature has in store.

Bad runs are excellent for training the mental aspects of the sport. Seize the opportunity to refine your ability to focus and get through tough stuff. Not all struggle should be avoided. Often, it can serve a purpose if you're willing to lean into it. Sometimes you have to let yourself suffer a bit to learn that you are capable of thriving under less than ideal circumstances.

Learn to Adapt

Sometimes you'll show up for a run and you just won't have what it takes to execute it as planned. Occasionally, the right answer isn't to push yourself through. In those instances, you have the opportunity to hone your ability to adapt and quickly shift gears to develop plan B on the fly.

Adaptability is mental agility. It's knowing when to pivot rather than just quit. It's the ability to take what's in front of you and work with it. In many ways, it's the acknowledgment that you understand that you won't always be able to show up as your very best self in every moment. Sometimes this means you shift your focus for the day or modify the workout, and other times it might mean that you walk away and try again tomorrow.

No matter how committed you are when you start your day, things can change. Life can be messy. At the time you set it, your running goal might have been really important to you, but your personal or professional priorities can change over the course of your training. Something else may actually become more important to you. This is why it's so important that you remember why you started. When conflicting priorities arise, your "why" becomes your touchstone. It's the thing you can look to in order to help you assess whether you need to push through the run or dedicate your energy elsewhere.

Without this periodic re-evaluation of your priorities, you might end up torn and chasing two things. You might end up feeling stuck, overwhelmed, and spread too thin if you prioritize too many things at once. Effort is only truly satisfying when it's channeled into the things that matter most to you, so you have to constantly be asking yourself what's most important.

This is yet another argument for being purposeful in the way you approach everything. When you know and understand the intention behind your running workout, it makes it easier to weigh your options and figure out whether to do the workout, modify the workout, or bag it. Absent a thoughtful consideration of the "why" behind what you're doing, it's difficult to make good decisions about how to proceed appropriately.

You have to begin with a plan to have direction; otherwise you wander aimlessly through life without purpose or improvement. But one thing is certain: not everything will go the way you've planned. The more prepared you are, the easier it becomes to navigate the times when unexpected things happen. Some days the victory is in just showing up and logging the miles. Other times, you'll have to adjust your focus for the workout, and in doing so you have the opportunity to get yourself a win regardless of your circumstances. Instead of simply scrapping the workout, you can choose to show up and define a mental training strategy for yourself that allows your training to continue in some way. Learn to pivot and carry on.

Believe You Can Improve

Over the years, I've worked with many people of different backgrounds, ages, and abilities. Among them all, one thing stands out as the clearest key indicator of success. It's not strength, talent, money, time, or skill. It's mindset. The people who think they can get better are the ones that do.

In her book *Mindset*, Carol Dweck talks about the fixed mindset—those who believe that the abilities each of us has are fixed and unchangeable—and the growth mindset—those who believe that abilities can be developed. In essence, growth-mindedness is the belief that you have the ability to change and grow; it's recognizing that where you are now is just the beginning. When a growth-minded individual tries to run a certain pace or distance and fails, she recognizes that she doesn't have the ability yet and then comes up with a plan to help her get there. Conversely, when a fixed-minded individual tries and fails, he assumes that the people who can do it are just more talented than he is and proceeds to make every excuse in the book for why he failed and will continue to fail.

It's a myth that some people are born with abilities that require no additional work to develop. History is full of stories of people who were widely acknowledged to be talented yet still fell short of reaching their full potential—perhaps because they leaned on their innate talent instead of developing it into something more. Talent will get you only so far. We all come into this world with different gifts, but that doesn't mean we stop there.

Any time you find yourself falling short, listen carefully to your own inner monologue. Does it sound like a fixed mindset, in which you believe things can't change and your ability level is final? If so, challenge yourself to consider how you could further develop your current abilities to get closer to where you want to be. Map out the road to improvement for yourself and remember that nothing is final. You're never stuck where you are unless you choose to be. If you can let go of all the excuses and complaints and instead focus on what you can do to move yourself forward, you just might find that the only thing holding you back is you.

Defining Success

The coolest part about developing mental durability is that it gives you the ability to define success for yourself. We've all had times in our lives where we've worked hard and gotten an extraordinary outcome that we're proud of, yet still technically fell short of what we initially set out to do. The skills laid out in this chapter are what enable such circumstances to occur.

The trick is realizing that you have the ability to define for yourself what success looks like every day. You have the power to choose whether you take it all in or focus on one area. You have the power to choose whether you push straight through the mess or whether you pivot. You have the power to choose your mindset.

Some days victory is in the small stuff. Other days it's much bigger. But you have the power and the responsibility to design your day in pursuit of the things that mean the most to you. And that's pretty awesome. The good news is that we each get to choose for ourselves how we measure our own effectiveness. The bad news is that most of us pick the wrong measurement tools.

When you begin, you have a goal that forms the target. If you judged your effectiveness based solely on whether you hit that target, the margin for error is small and there's no accounting for the unexpected and uncontrollable. In looking solely to goal-fulfillment as a measurement of success, you place your ability to succeed partially out of your own control. You never want to be in a position where your success hinges not on you but on your circumstances.

Rather than leaving it all to chance, I propose that—instead of judging your success based on whether you hit a specific target somewhere down the line—you focus on the quality of work you put into it. Gauge your effectiveness based on your effort not the results. Instead of "Did I achieve a new 10K PR?" ask "Did I put everything I had into maximizing my training time?" Instead of "Did I hit my splits?" ask yourself "Did I consistently refuse to let myself fade in the final 400 meters of each repeat?" In doing so, you put the power to succeed back where it belongs: in your own hands.

The road to improvement is long. It's easy to fall into the trap of being short-sighted and treating each training run like it's pass/fail. Progress is often not linear. Sometimes you have to do a little worse today in order to be better down the road. Remember that you're not failing as long as you're practicing something of value.

For my sixth ultramarathon, I trained all winter long in the snow, ice, freezing temps, and lots of sleet. My paces through training were right on target and I felt strong as I finished my final long run three weeks out from race day—I was ready to bag myself a shiny new PR. Then, two days before the race, the seasons changed—from winter directly into summer. On race day, the temps reached nearly 100 degrees with 90% humidity. I had a choice: get bent out shape about not being able to PR this race or go out there and give it everything I've got. To this day, finishing that race in those conditions (without having to visit the medic tent) is one of my proudest moments—even though it was my slowest 50K time. You always have a choice about how you move through less than ideal circumstances and define success for yourself. You can let your training efforts go to waste or you can go out there and find a way to make yourself proud regardless.

KEY POINT: *Motivation*

The most frequently asked question I get about training is "How do you stay motivated?" The short answer is: you don't. But here's the good news—you don't have to have motivation to get things done.

The reality is that motivation is fleeting. In order to be durable enough to carry on, you have to be committed to your goals and the process it takes to get there. I talk to many runners who want to qualify for the Boston Marathon and get all hyped up to try, but they aren't fully aware of what that process entails—or worse, they aren't being honest with themselves about whether they're able to do the things required to get them there. Then, when the wheels fall of the wagon, they cry "lack of motivation," when the true lack was committing to the process no matter what.

Instead of waiting for motivation to grace you with her presence, focus on creating habits. If you create a habit, you have something to lean on when you're not feeling motivated. Habits are the mechanisms that allow you to focus on the daily discipline of the process (like your effort) rather than the end goal (like the result). Create the habit and stick to it no matter what. Some days you might show up and do poorly, but you win because you didn't break the chain of habit. You don't have to be motivated. Be committed.

Also, what often registers intellectually as lack of motivation could really be a recovery issue. Runners often cite a lack of energy as the main reason they aren't taking steps to reach their running goals. While these are legitimate complaints, I ask, "What are you doing about that?" If your day drains you, what are you doing to recharge? If you're always tired, what steps are you taking to get more sleep? If your schedule is packed, what are you willing to take off your plate to free up space for yourself? While it's easy and convenient to say you don't have the time or energy, you're really only selling yourself short. If you don't like the situation you're in, it's up to you to change it.

Dealing with Pressure

I once heard someone define pressure as the belief that you have to go harder, faster, and better than you think you're capable of. And when you frame it like that, it becomes easier to understand why pressure is a part of the process of improvement. In order to get better, you have to be living at the edge of your current capabilities—you do this intentionally because you know that you don't improve by doing the things that are already comfortable to you. Adaptation occurs only in the fringes, when we stretch ourselves just beyond our current capabilities.

By signing on for growth and development, you are signing on for pressure. You do this because the thing you want is on the other side of it. So when the pressure is mounting and your hands are getting sweaty and your stomach is in knots, it helps to remember that you chose it. In that moment, you can see that pressure as an obstacle or a rite of passage.

Remember why you're doing this in the first place. I'm willing to accept suffering when it's for something that matters to me. Look for purpose in the struggle and remind yourself that you're choosing that path with the goal of being a better version of yourself. When you're motivated by a specific purpose, it's typically easier to sacrifice immediate gratification for long-term gain.

Once your purpose is clear and your head is on straight again, lean into the challenge. The road to improvement leads you right up to the line between what you can handle right now and the next level up. It's supposed to be hard. It's supposed to be uncomfortable. If it's not, it's not doing anything to help you get better.

Changing Your Relationship with Failure

Because the name of this game is playing at your edge in terms of what makes you stronger and what makes you feel like you're breaking down, know that it's inevitable that at some point you will miscalculate and fail. But failure is just feedback. It's a sign that you're not there yet. It may even give you valuable information about where your abilities are lacking and illuminate your untapped potential.

Expect that at some point you will feel the sting of disappointment.

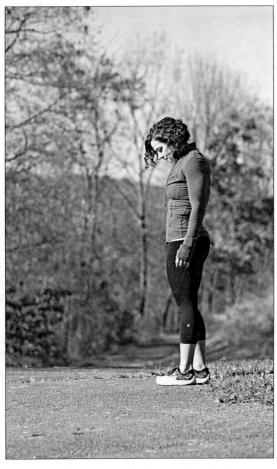

Failure is simply a form of feedback.

No amount of planning, training, or strategizing will save you from that. The only way around it is to set your expectations so low that you can't fail—but there is no fulfillment or joy to be found there. The pain that comes from living in fear of failure is much worse and lasts much longer than the actual failure could ever be.

In that space where you accept failure as a normal and necessary part of growth and move on, durability is born. Learning to hold both your frustration and your desire for growth at the same time is no easy task—they seem at odds and want to pull you in different directions. But you can be both disappointed and willing to try again—it's not a choice you have to make. This dissatisfaction you feel can be powerful if you develop a good relationship with it. When you learn that and move forward, your resilience grows.

Failure is feedback you'll inevitably receive—we all do. Don't read anything more into it than you've still got work to do. This is not your final destination. Use the experience to learn how to tweak your training or better read your own gauge. When you can face the day with humility and be willing to see where you still have room to grow, suddenly your struggle today can no longer define who you'll be tomorrow.

Making a Comeback

When things go wrong, and they do for all of us at some point, it's important to know how to bring yourself back. Disappointment can quickly turn into a black hole, a downward spiral that leaves you questioning, "Am I enough?" I've been there. Odds are you have too.

You are entitled to your emotions. It's a normal part of investing so much of yourself into something. You're upset about it because it was something that mattered to you. Feel the feelings. Let them wash over you and knock you down. But don't stay there.

That's where some people get stuck—buried under a pile of self-pity, paralyzed by the fear of having to feel the pain of failure again. In doing so, these people have given that failure power over what happens next, and the path forward disappears. Your circumstances are merely the starting point for what happens next. Accept the feedback that failure handed you and focus on your next move. Look for things that you control—they may be few, but I promise they're there.

The quicker you're able to sift through everything and identify what you control, the faster you'll find your way out of the mess. Don't forget that you always have a choice. You have a choice in the way you endure the challenges in your life. You have a choice about your attitude. You have a choice about how you support yourself through the struggle. That's where your power lies: in recognizing that you don't control everything, but you control something—and in the end, that something is the only thing that really matters.

My own potential as a runner would never have been fully realized if I'd let the setbacks I faced along the way take me off track. All my major running accomplishments, including every ultramarathon I've ever completed, came after numerous injuries and a hip fracture. I'm glad I never gave up. But more importantly, I'm glad that I didn't waste the time I spent injured sitting around and feeling sorry for myself—thinking about what might have been. In-

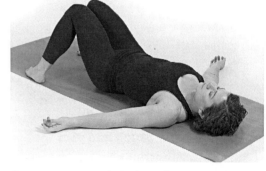

Constructive rest breathing https://youtu.be/ kUmOzNgN3dA

stead, I spent the time improving the links in the chain that would ensure I came back stronger. I put the wheels in motion as best I could and in the process I paved the way for myself to get out of the mess.

Don't let yourself get lost in the frustration. Pay attention to the right things. Ask yourself, "In this moment, what do I control?" Don't waste your energy fighting with the rest of it.

KEY POINT:
A Breathing Exercise for When You're Feeling Overwhelmed

We've all had to wrestle with a feeling of being suffocating or crushed. In those times, the words of support you receive from those around you and even the words in this chapter may not do anything to lessen the feeling that the walls are closing in on you. The only thing you can do in those moments is breathe. Everything you think and feel in your life is temporary. It helps to soften your resistance to what you're experiencing so that it can pass.

Try this simple breathing exercise when you're overwhelmed.

1. Set a timer for five minutes (or more if you have it).

2. Lie on your back with your knees bent and your feet flat on the floor. Separate your feet so they are slightly wider than your hips and let your knees fall in and rest on each other.

3. Rest your hands comfortably either on your belly or on the floor and add a blanket if you'd prefer something under your head. You're looking for a position that requires no effort and is easy to drop into so that you can let your body lean into the floor and be really passive.

4. First, just notice your breath and let it move naturally. Without trying to lengthen or deepen your breath, count how long it takes you to inhale—this might be a count of three, four, or five. The pace of your count doesn't matter as long as it's a consistent cadence throughout the exercise.

5. After you've established how long it takes you to inhale in a relaxed way, start to draw out and lengthen your exhales to match the count of your inhales. So if you were inhaling for a count of

four, slowly extend your exhales to a count of four to match the length of your inhales.

6. After a few rounds of breath with equal length inhales and exhales, gradually start to lengthen your exhales by a count of one or two more than your inhales. So if you were inhaling and exhaling for a count of four, you'd extend your exhales to a count of five or six.

7. Your breathing should be relaxed throughout. Stick with a count that doesn't make you feel like you need to grip or tense to maintain the breath count.

8. If at any point your mind wanders and you lose the count, gently bring yourself back to the count. The goal isn't never to lose count, it's to keep coming back every time you drift away from it.

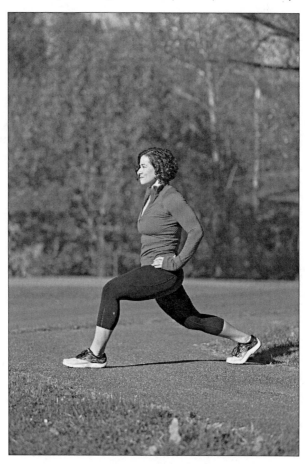

Practice makes habit.

Everything Is Practice

We are all capable of growth and change. But things don't just change on their own. You have to practice changing them. Every choice, every habit, every day matters because it's all practice. In every moment of your life you are practicing something. If you're not practicing being different than you were yesterday, then you're practicing being the same. You have to practice being the person you want to be. You have to practice being mentally durable the way you practice your track intervals and hill repeats.

You have to work at developing your mental skills the way you work at developing your physical abilities. Like everything else we've covered in this book, it takes a lot of exploration and self-evaluation to figure out. You've got to be brutally honest with yourself about what isn't coming as naturally to you. And then you have to be willing to confront it. If it matters to you, you have to work at it.

The only way to get anywhere—in running or in life—is to start where you are, decide where you want to go, and the steps necessary to move yourself in that direction. One step at a time, one breath at a time, one mile at a time, one choice at a time.

Part 6: The Big Picture

Now that you've seen the constituent parts of durability, let's find the best ways to use and apply this information in real time and real life.

Your personal durability plan should be based on the movements and work that you find most challenging for you or less familiar because those will ultimately be the most beneficial. The two basic approaches that I use for myself and my athletes are to (1) use some of the activation work as a pre-run warm-up circuit and (2) use some mobility work and SMR to create a straight-up recovery session.

These are simply examples of how you take the work prescribed in this book and create a practice that best supports you and your goals. In the next chapter, we'll look at some more individualized ways you can incorporate this work into your life; here, we'll see how to use these durability tools before and after your run.

Pre-Run Warm-Up Circuit

When I was writing this book, I'd spend the better part of the day most days of the week at my desk researching, writing, editing, and otherwise fussing around with the content. Inevitably, my body would start to complain and I'd feel the urge to go for a run. But after spending hours sitting with less-than-stellar computer posture, my body wasn't really ready for just lacing up my shoes and heading out the door. I tried once or twice, and it made the first two miles more miserable than they needed to be.

Posture during the day and even how you slept last night can impact your readiness to run well. Sometimes your body could use a little help before you force it from one long-held position to upright movement. The practice that follows is what I use to unwind the tension from sitting at my desk and fire up the muscles that tend to spend the day underutilized. After this quick warm-up, I'm out the door feeling good rather than stiff, sloppy, and fatigued. This circuit also works well if you run first thing in the morning to get your running muscles primed for movement.

I recommend doing this quick circuit two to three times through. I prefer to do it without shoes to help activate the muscles of my feet and toes, but it can also be done with shoes.

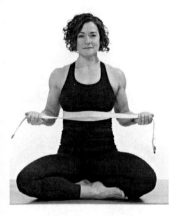

Seated Strap Breathing (page 113).

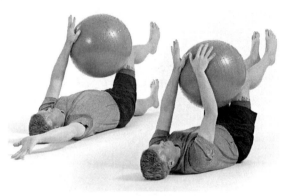

Stability Ball Dead Bug (page 121).

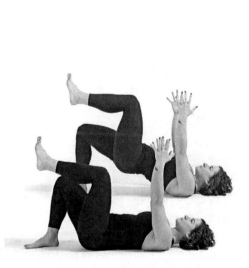

Single Leg Bridges (page 97).

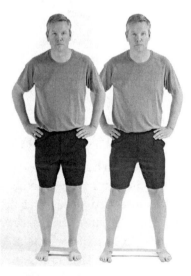

Foot Banded Lateral Walks (page 99).

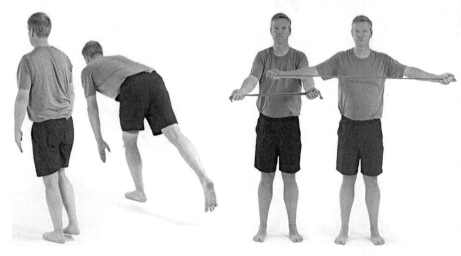

Single Leg Deadlifts (page 100).   Resistance Band Pull Aparts (page 147).

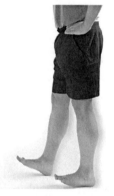 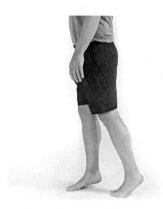

Heel Walking (page 68).   Ball of Foot Walking (page 68).

Straight-Up Recovery Session

As you train, race, and push yourself to your limits, you also occasionally must shut everything down in order to allow the systems of your body to recover, adapt, and catch up to the demands you're placing on them. You get stronger in the recovery time between workouts, not in the workouts themselves. It's easy to take for granted the healing processes that occur at the cellular level in your body. You might think that the passage of time alone will be enough to get you ready to face the next stressor. Often it's not.

You have to be an active participant in your own recovery and healing. The best way to do that is to simply create space for stillness and silence. When you do that, you're giving your nervous system time to sink into relaxation mode so that your body can do what it's naturally good at—remodeling, healing, circulating, and digesting. You have a role to play in directing the internal chemistry that's always working inside you. In these moments of stillness and silence, your body can direct its energy resources away from doing, thinking, and achieving. Instead, it can focus on maintaining the systems that keep you going by rebuilding and repairing.

The recovery practice that follows is designed to stimulate those systems by creating space for stillness and silence while helping to restore full range of motion to your joints. It's amazing what your body can do and how quickly the inner chemistry can change when you consciously take time to let the systems work and support you. It's also a fabulous way to wind down and recover from weekly long runs.

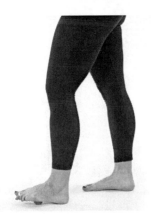

Feet SMR (page 63).

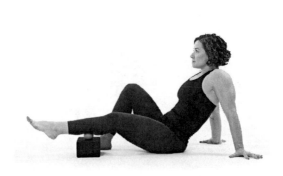

Calves SMR (page 64).

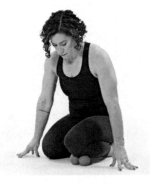

Shins SMR (page 65).

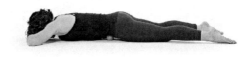

Iliopsoas SMR (page 119).

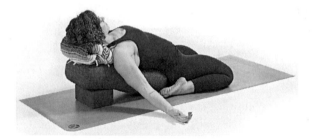

Supported Saddle (page 85).

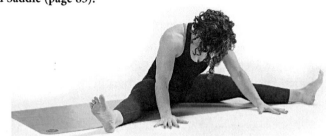

Supported Straddle (page 86).

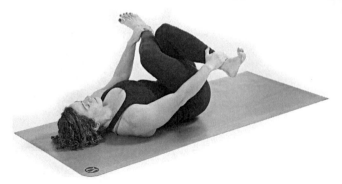

Reclined Cross-Legged Stretch (page 89).

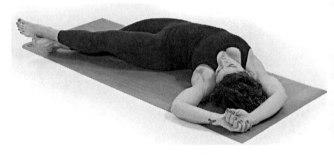

Banana (page 116).

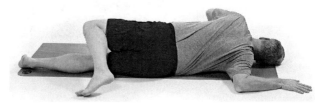

Prone Cactus Stretch (page 139).

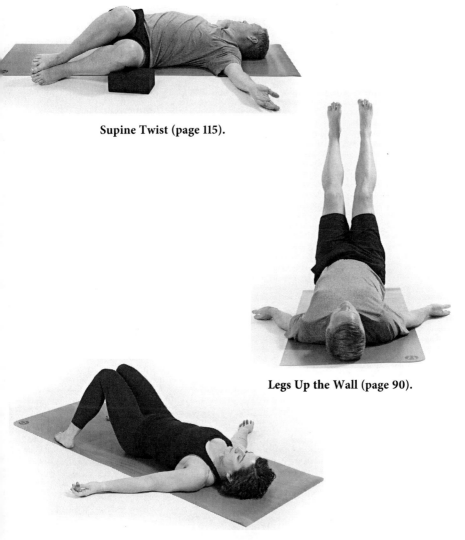

Supine Twist (page 115).

Legs Up the Wall (page 90).

Extended Exhalation Breathing (page 169).

Maintenance Schedule: Creating a Routine That Works

You should not treat your body like a machine—it's far more complex, dynamic, and responsive than even the fanciest sports car. However, there's definitely an argument to be made for maintaining your body in accordance with a schedule. As an athlete, you demand a lot from your body and subject it to the regular stress of training. My goal is to get you spending just a little more time tending to its needs.

In this chapter, I'll answer some frequently asked questions and outline ways that you can use the material in this book to develop a routine maintenance schedule for yourself that's tailored to your specific areas of concern to create whole-body durability.

How Do I Create a Routine That Works for Me?

There really aren't any rules here. We are all unique individuals with different goals, habits, and abilities. Because of that, it's not an easy question to answer. But there are many right answers and hardly any wrong ones. This book is full of simple ideas to get you started on figuring out what works best for you and your life. It's up to you to invest the time and effort into figuring out which of the stretches, SMR techniques, and exercises make you and your body feel better. Then focus your time, energy, and efforts there in order to create the biggest impact. If you're already working with a physical therapist, corrective exercise specialist, or yoga teacher who knows your personal history, it might be beneficial for you to show them this book and let them help guide you on the best ways to create a routine that works for you.

How Much Time Should I Spend in Each Session? And How Often?

The sample practices I provided for you in the preceding chapter vary in terms of length. You don't need to dedicate large chunks of time to your durability training in order to reap the benefits. Work with the time you have. If you have 20 minutes, four times per week, that's great—spend two of those days working on corrective work and the other two on mobility and SMR. If you have 15 minutes every day, you can totally work with that, too—alternate daily between corrective work, mobility, and SMR based on what your running schedule has in store for you each day. Here are a few ways that have worked well for my clients:

Five Days of Running with Five Days of Durability Training

Monday	Tuesday	Wednesday	Thursday	Friday	Saturday	Sunday
	Track Intervals	Easy Run	Tempo Run		Easy Run	Long Run (AM)
30 minutes of mobility and SMR*		30 minutes of corrective strength work*		30 minutes of mobility and SMR*	30 minutes of corrective strength work*	Straight-Recovery Practice (PM)

Four Days of Running with Two Days of Strength Training and Seven Days of Durability Training

Monday	Tuesday	Wednesday	Thursday	Friday	Saturday	Sunday
Strength Training	Easy Run	Strength Training	Track Intervals	Easy Run	Long Run	Rest
Warm-up with 15 minutes of corrective strength work**	15 minutes of hip and core SMR work***	Warm-up with 15 minutes of corrective strength work**	15 minutes of foot, lower leg, and hip mobility work***	Warm-up with 15 minutes of corrective strength work**	20 minutes of foot, lower leg, and shoulder SMR work***	45 minutes of total body mobility work

*Select two to four helpful movements from each section of this book to perform.

**Select one or two helpful movements from each section of this book and perform them in a quick circuit.

***Set a timer, select a few movements to do from each of the specified sections of this book, and work through them until time is up.

My personal preference is to favor frequency over duration. I can usually find an extra 15 minutes in my day, but a whole hour is much harder to make happen. It's easier for me to break up the work into small chunks and sprinkle them in throughout the week. I always make sure to dedicate a few minutes per day before each of my workouts to work on mobility and SMR in the areas that I know tend to be chronically tighter in my body—like my right side iliopsoas, right side piriformis, and all the muscles of my quads on both sides. I also focus a few minutes per day on other areas that feel tense or that I've been working particularly hard that week. Before all my runs and strength training workouts, I include a few corrective strengthening exercises into my warm-up and some mobility work in my cool-down.

When I first started training for durability, I was chronically injured and had a lot going on in my body that needed to be addressed. Initially, I dedicated more time every week to building durability. Once things in my body started to feel better and the injuries subsided, I had to do a lot less work every week to maintain durability. What started out as an hour, six days per week, is now more like 15–30 minutes per day. I also spend more time on durability training when I'm not actively training for a race and I gradually reduce the time as the mileage increases since there are only so many hours in the day.

What Should I Focus On?

It's not necessary for you to do all the work in this book. You might try it out at first to see what you find most helpful, but eventually you'll narrow the scope and end up with a much shorter list of exercises, stretches, and techniques that really seem to make you feel better after you've done them. Remember that the goal is to get to know yourself and your body's needs better in order to move closer toward balance, so it's not necessary for you to focus your time and energy resources on the things that feel easy for you or don't seem to have any effect on how you or your body feels. I'd rather you dedicate your time to doing the things that actually move the dial for you. This means you'll have to spend time focusing on things that don't come as easily for you, and that can be hard on your ego. But you have to ask yourself: do I want to feel good, or do I want to feel better?

What's the Best Way to Fit It into My Day?

No program in the world, regardless of how innovative or brilliant it is, will help you if you can't actually fit the work into your life and execute it consistently. So I tell my clients that the easiest way to start incorporating this work into your routine is by identifying pockets of time that you already have and/or could use more effectively. For example, if you tend to hang out in your living room in the evening and watch television with your significant other or kids, use some of that time to do some SMR or light mobility work on the floor. Or if you have the habit of waking up and mindlessly scrolling through social media in the morning, use some of that time to do corrective strength work instead to get your day started out right. Once you start to see the compounded effects of including this work in your life, it becomes easier to set aside more time.

Can I Do These Exercises on My Running Days?

If your run training is divided up among harder effort days (like intervals, hill repeats, long run, etc.) and easier effort days, remember to keep your easy days easy. If you're not on a specific training plan with hard and easy days, anything goes. Just remember to give yourself ample rest and some easier-effort days every week. See the charts on page 180 for some ideas and options for making it work.

Rest days and easy days are good days to do some mobility work and SMR—nothing strenuous, because the focus is on recovery. Also, some light mobility work and SMR can feel really great later in the day after your long runs to help you unwind and open up the range of motion in your joints after logging all those miles.

As far as when to incorporate the corrective strength work, it depends on how your body responds to the corrective strengthening work. Although many of the movements in this book appear mild, know that the first few times you do them, you might notice some muscle soreness in the days after—perhaps even muscles you've never felt in the past. Remember, we're working deep to activate and strengthen the stabilizer muscles, so don't be surprised when things start waking up. Unless you've not been doing anything other than running in the past few years, you should not be substantially sore after the workouts. Once you know how the corrective work prescribed in this book affects you, you can use a few of the movements as a pre-run warm-up before your harder-effort runs or include a few of the movements on your easier-effort days to keep the blood flowing and your muscles active.

What If I'm Already Strength Training?

First of all, awesome. Keep that up—strength training will go a long way toward helping you become more durable. If you're already strength training, it's pretty simple to slot the work you find most beneficial from this book into the early stages of your warm-up before tackling your main sets. Then, once you're done with your strength training workout, cool down and unwind with some mobility work or SMR, which feel really great after lifting.

What About In-Season Training Versus Off-Season Training?

If you're a runner that has distinct periods of the year where you are "in season"—that is, building mileage and training at higher intensity for races—and other times when you're in your "off season" with the focus on simply maintaining your base level of fitness, you can set up your durability training to align with your seasons. In your off season, spend more time devoted to establishing greater total-body durability, which can carry you through your next training cycle. Then, while in season, shift your focus to race-specific training and do shorter durability training sessions throughout the week to maintain the work you did during your off season.

Your Self-Care Is Your Responsibility

The approach I've presented in this book is the same as what I recommend to all my clients and students—be honest about where you are now and take stock of your injuries, habits, patterns, repetitive movements, and postural considerations. Then decide what you want to change, identify the steps you need to move in the direction you want to go, and practice constantly.

Don't get so reliant on your teachers and coaches to tell you what to do that you forget to pay attention to what your mind and body actually need. If your goal is to run well, move well, and be well for life, you have to know how to do this for yourself and be willing to take care of yourself. No one knows you better than you, and no one is ultimately responsible for the decisions you make about how you spend your time but you. Others may guide you, but the person you're ultimately accountable to is yourself.

This will be a lifelong process. As with all good things in life, there are no shortcuts or quick fixes. But you are and always will be a worthwhile investment. And you always have some say in where you go from here.

Resources

Find exclusive bonus content at www.alisonheilig.com/thedurable runnerbook.

Recommended Equipment

RAD Rounds and Recovery Rounds
www.radroller.com

Perform Better Superbands and Mini Bands
www.performbetter.com

Recommended Reading

The Athlete's Guide to Yoga by Sage Rountree (VeloPress, 2008)
NASM Essentials of Corrective Exercise Training, edited by Michael A. Clark, Scott C. Lucett, and Brian G. Sutton (Jones and Bartlett Learning, 2014)

Index

Numbers in *bold italics* indicate pages with illustrations

187